Snacking Habits
for
Healthy Living

The American Dietetic Association

JOHN WILEY & SONS, INC.

New York • Chichester • Weinheim • Brisbane • Singapore • Toronto

Snacking Habits for Healthy Living: Up-to-Date Tips from the World's Foremost Nutrition Experts. © 1997 by The American Dietetic Association.

This book is printed on acid-free paper. ⊖

Library of Congress Cataloging-in-Publication Data

Snacking habits for healthy living / The American Dietetic Association

   p.   cm.
Includes index.

ISBN 0-471-34704-3

Edited by: Jeff Braun
Cover Design: Terry Dugan Design
Text Design & Production: David Enyeart
Art/Production Manager: Claire Lewis

10   9   8   7   6

Snacking Habits
for
Healthy Living

Written for The American Dietetic Association by
Jean Storlie, MS, RD
JS Associates, Inc.
Ithaca, New York

The American Dietetic Association Reviewers:
Corrine Bronson-Adatto,
MS, RD, FADA
Highland Park, Illinois

Eleese Cunningham, RD
National Center for Nutrition
and Dietetics
Chicago, Illinois

Marilyn Lawler, PhD, RD
University of Chicago Hospitals
Chicago, Illinois

Technical Editor:
Betsy Hornick, MS, RD
The American Dietetic Association
Chicago, Illinois

THE AMERICAN DIETETIC ASSOCIATION is the largest group of food and nutrition professionals in the world. As the advocate of the profession, the ADA serves the public by promoting optimal nutrition, health, and well-being.

For expert answers to your nutrition questions, call the ADA/National Center for Nutrition and Dietetics Hot Line at (900) 225-5267. To listen to recorded messages or obtain a referral to an RD in your area, call (800) 366-1655.

Table of Contents

Introduction

WHEN WAS THE LAST TIME you skipped breakfast and lunch, arrived home famished, and snacked steadily until bedtime? Do you ever snack in response to stress or boredom? How often do you snack while watching television or surfing the net? Do you mindlessly munch on snacks while chatting at parties? Chances are you answered "yes" to at least one of these questions. Most would probably agree—we are a nation of snackers.

For some of us, such as young children, teenagers, and athletes, snacking is important for meeting calorie and nutrient needs, while others may need to modify snacking habits to curtail fat and calorie intake. Experts agree that snacking habits should be considered—not necessarily eliminated—when building a healthy diet. Read on for more on making the most out of your snacking habits.

Grazing Your Way to Health

As our lifestyles become more hectic, many of us lack the time and consistent schedules to sit down and eat three "square" meals. In fact, about 40 percent of Americans eat four or more meals a day, many of which are grabbed on the run. This eating pattern of munching and crunching throughout the day is often referred to as "grazing." Grazers eat on the run, eat small amounts more often, and often eat independently of other family members.

Grazing can be an effective way of filling in the extra calories and nutrients that would otherwise be missing from small or skipped meals. But grazing also can be a source of extra calories, fat, and salt—nutrients that most people need to moderate. If you think of snacks as mini-meals that serve as building blocks to a healthy diet instead of extra treats, grazing can be a healthy style of eating. And for some, it is also a more convenient way to eat.

Eating several well-balanced mini-meals a day can help to:

Optimize your energy and mental power. Going more than 4 hours without eating deprives you of the fuel needed to concentrate and function at your best.

Control your weight. Eating at frequent intervals prevents you from becoming too hungry, which in turn makes it easier to keep from overeating.

Reduce the load on your heart. After you eat, your heart pumps extra blood to your stomach and intestines to help digest the meal—the larger the meal, the more work for your heart. (For example, in the two hours following a 240-calorie meal, the heart pumps an extra 84 quarts of blood and an extra 258 quarts following a 720-calorie meal.)

Prevent heartburn. Large meals are more likely to cause stomach acids to reflux into the esophagus causing heartburn.

Snack Food Trends

As we grab for snacks, three factors drive our choices: taste, health, and convenience. In fact, taste is cited most often as the reason why certain between-meal treats are selected. The most popular snacks are salty and crunchy. They rank third among all foods in total super-market sales and account for 20 percent of daily calories. These snacks are usually eaten in the afternoon and evening. Because so many of us crave sweet and chocolate flavors, it's not surprising that baked goods and candy follow salty/crunchy foods in popularity. When it comes to choosing snacks for good health, fruit and other fresh snacks are becoming more popular. Children and older adults prefer fruit for a morning snack, while middle-aged adults are more likely to select baked goods.

The entire food industry is responding to the snacking habits and health consciousness of Americans. Today's nutrition savvy snack-ers have more and more choices. Old favorites like chips, crackers, and cookies are now available in lower fat and, for some, fat-free versions. You can also find foods portioned for snacking: bagel bites, miniature stuffed pocket sandwiches, and pizza rolls to name a few. Snack packs containing fresh vegetables, low-fat dip, and pretzels or breadsticks appeal to on-the-go consumers looking for a convenient and healthy snack or mini-meal. Packaging also caters to the increase in snacking. Pudding, jello, applesauce, yogurt, cottage cheese, and canned fruit are now packaged in single-serve, snack-friendly containers.

With time constraints afflicting most everyone's lifestyle, it's no wonder that convenience plays a key role in many food choices. Retail stores have recognized that today's snackers care about nutrition as well as convenience. Some stores now feature a healthy snack section, others create healthful snacking displays throughout the store to attract health-conscious customers. A common merchandising tactic in convenience stores is to place hot-selling snacks together, creating tie-ins of foods that go together. For example, you'll find salty snacks next to the beverage cooler. Gourmet coffee drinkers will find bakery snacks nearby. For the "jog in" traffic, sports drinks and sports bars are displayed side by side. Although some of these tie-ins can be a money and calorie trap, they support the concept of making snacks "mini-meals."

A Lifestyle Approach

This book is intended to show you how to make snacking a healthy part of your lifestyle. Keep these guidelines in mind as you develop snacking habits for healthy living:

Snacks are building blocks of a healthy diet. Think of your snack food choices as important pieces in a puzzle that makes up a healthy eating pattern—they are more than the "icing on the cake."

All foods can fit. There are no right or wrong snack foods. All foods can be part of a healthful eating style when consumed in moderation and balanced over one or more days.

Moderation is the key to making all foods fit. Most Americans can benefit from moderating how often and how much they eat of foods containing high levels of calories, fat, salt, and sugar.

Variety is the spice of life. Selecting snack foods from a variety of food groups is key to meeting nutritional needs. Besides, variety lends pleasure and interest to eating.

Healthful snacking tastes great! Eating delicious food is one of life's great pleasures.

Chapter 1, "Building Blocks of Healthy Snacking," covers the basics of healthy snacking. This information applies to snackers of every age and situation. Because it serves as a springboard for the issues addressed in later chapters, you'll want to be familiar with the information discussed in Chapter 1 before delving into the later chapters.

Chapters 2 through 5 deal with the nutrition and snacking needs for specific groups of people: children, teenagers, athletes, and weight-conscious adults. The special nutritional needs of these individuals are well-suited to a style of eating that includes regular snacks.

Chapters 6 through 8 address situations and settings where Americans typically snack: at work, at home, and on the go. Practical guidelines and strategies are provided for making these snacking situations a healthy part of your lifestyle. You may find that only one or all of these situations apply to your snacking habits.

Snacking is very important for those with health or disease conditions that create special nutrition needs. Chapter 9, "Special Snacking Needs," addresses the snacking needs of people with diabetes or hypoglycemia, and those who need to gain weight. These groups are not the only ones with special dietary needs. However, snacking plays an important role in dietary management of these conditions.

The appendices include specific ideas and guidelines for snack food choices. Appendix A contains lists of snack foods organized by food group and includes the amounts of certain nutrients to guide your choices. Appendix B presents guidelines for selecting snacks from each food group, including the key nutrients, lower fat and lower calorie choices, higher fat and higher calorie choices, and tips for healthy and convenient snacking. Appendix C provides ideas for satisfying sensory cravings with lower fat and lower calorie snacks. Use these appendices in conjunction with the information in the individual chapters to select snacks, develop shopping lists, and create snack food stashes at home, work, and anywhere you snack.

Snacking can be a habit that nourishes and sustains you—or a source of excess calories and fat. How you fit snacking into your life is a personal choice. Read on to discover the joys of healthy snacking.

Chapter One

Building Blocks of Healthy Snacking

ONCE CONSIDERED EXTRA TREATS, eaten above and beyond three square meals, snacking has taken on a new meaning. Snacking today comprises a significant portion of the total calories consumed by many people and touches many aspects of our lives. Whether this translates to a healthy eating style depends on your attitudes toward snacking, your snack food choices, and how snacking fits into your overall diet. This chapter lays the foundation for healthy snacking, starting with a self-assessment of your snacking habits. Helpful tools for building a healthy diet, such as the Food Guide Pyramid and the Nutrition Facts label, are presented to help you construct a healthy approach to snacking. And to keep you on track with the facts, common myths about snacking are dispelled.

Why Do You Snack?

People snack for many reasons. For some, snacking is the most convenient way to eat—hectic schedules don't accommodate sit-down meals. For others, snacking stems from habits and routines developed over the years, like munching in front of the TV set or nibbling while cooking. Still others snack in response to emotions. Sadness, boredom, anxiety, and loneliness are common triggers for snacking, but joyful and happy feelings also can signal an opportunity to indulge. Understanding why you snack is an important first step in making your snacking habits part of healthy living. Complete the following snacking habits profile to identify the reasons why you snack.

Your Snacking Habits

Check off (✔) all the reasons why you snack. Then add up the number of responses in each section.

I snack when I...

Section 1

- ❏ feel hungry
- ❏ eat dinner late
- ❏ miss lunch
- ❏ feel lightheaded and tired
- ❏ eat a light breakfast
- ❏ am too busy to eat a meal
- ❏ miss breakfast
- ❏ hear my stomach grumbling
- ❏ eat a light lunch
- ❏ eat a light dinner

___ **Total**

Section 2

- ❏ feel bored
- ❏ feel stressed out
- ❏ need comfort
- ❏ feel lonely
- ❏ have a hard day at work
- ❏ feel anxious
- ❏ feel joyful, excited
- ❏ feel frustrated
- ❏ need to lift my spirits
- ❏ feel like celebrating

___ **Total**

Section 3

- ❏ am offered snacks
- ❏ talk on the phone
- ❏ am watching TV
- ❏ see food that tastes good
- ❏ am preparing food
- ❏ go to parties
- ❏ am in the car
- ❏ am at my desk
- ❏ see someone else snacking
- ❏ am avoiding something unpleasant

___ **Total**

Which section had the largest number of check marks?

Section 1: You snack because of a physical need for food. If you snack because you're hungry or too busy to stop for a meal, then snacks play an important role in meeting your need for food—they should be part of your daily meal plan. Plan ahead for snacks rather than grabbing food impulsively. Think of snacks as mini-meals and coordinate them into your overall diet.

Section 2: Emotional triggers may be influencing your snacking habits; these triggers often lead to overeating. If you snack to relieve stress or boredom, then snacking can become a problem. These snacking routines often lead to overeating and can be difficult to break. Seek other emotional outlets, such as talking to a friend or going for a walk. If you munch to satisfy your need to crunch and chew, grab foods like carrots, celery, and pretzels which offer a lot of crunch but few calories.

Section 3: Habits and unconscious behaviors are playing a key role in why you snack; these routines often result in overeating. If your snacking accompanies other activities and behaviors, try making some substitutions. Either swap eating for a new activity, or substitute lower calorie foods. For example, knit or do some kind of handwork while watching TV. Or replace potato chips with air- or stove-popped popcorn, cookies with fresh fruit, ice cream with low-fat frozen yogurt or sherbet.

Building Healthy Snacking Habits

Look at your lifestyle and identify which times of the day you are likely to go for more than 3 to 4 hours between eating. Think about what is happening during these times; it's possible that you're faced with time constraints and limited food choices. Then think creatively about new approaches. What foods could you pack or stash so that you don't get stuck high and dry? Review the foods listed in Appendix A and identify which foods will work for you. Use the accompanying information in Appendix B to help you tailor the choices to fit your lifestyle. If your snack choices are influenced by sensory cravings, such as for salty, sweet, crunchy or chewy foods, the ideas listed in Appendix C may be helpful.

Healthy Snacking Tips

Spread your snacks throughout the day; try not to do all your snacking in the evening.

Use snacks to fill the nutritional gaps in your diet.

Be aware that adding snacks on top of your usual diet may lead to weight gain.

Surround yourself with healthy snacks—stash them in your refrigerator, desk drawer, briefcase, backpack, gym bag, and car.

Watch your portion sizes—many snacks are easy to overeat. Single-serve containers can help you keep portions in check.

Building Blocks of Healthy Snacking

The following strategies are building blocks for healthy snacking:

Treat snacks as mini-meals. When you view snacks as an integral part of your daily diet, each snack becomes a mini-meal, rather than an empty-calorie item, which contains calories but few nutrients. By combining traditional snack foods, such as chips or cookies, with foods from other food groups, you can improve the nutritional value of your snack. For example, serving apple slices and nonfat milk with graham crackers to your children for an afternoon snack provides 30 percent of the daily need for calcium and 16 percent of both the vitamin C and fiber requirement. Adding half a green and half a red pepper to a snack of salsa and tortilla chips boosts the vitamin C level to 130 percent and vitamin A to 15 percent of the recommended intake. To turn a snack into a mini-meal, combine foods from different food groups, rather than eating just a single food.

Let the Pyramid guide your choices. Build your snacks around the concepts of balance, variety, and moderation. The Food Guide Pyramid illustrates how you can achieve these goals. To balance your nutrient intake, eat more snacks from the base of the Pyramid (grains, fruits, and vegetables) and go easy on the foods at the tip (fats, oils, and sweets). Fats, oils, and sweets add pleasure to eating but contain mostly calories and/or fat with few nutrients, so you'll want to moderate your intake of these foods. If your favorite foods are high in fat and calories, the key is balancing how often and how much you eat of these foods.

Food Guide Pyramid

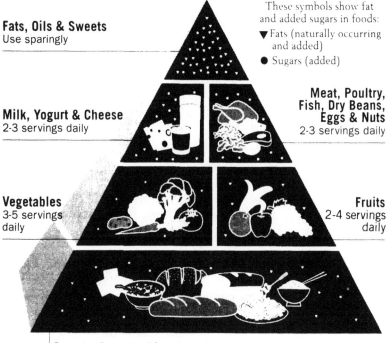

Fats, Oils & Sweets
Use sparingly

These symbols show fat and added sugars in foods:
▼ Fats (naturally occurring and added)
● Sugars (added)

Milk, Yogurt & Cheese
2-3 servings daily

Meat, Poultry, Fish, Dry Beans, Eggs & Nuts
2-3 servings daily

Vegetables
3-5 servings daily

Fruits
2-4 servings daily

Breads, Cereals, Rice & Pasta
6-11 servings daily

Calorie Levels

1,600: About right for many sedentary women and some older adults

2,200: About right for most children, teenage girls, active women, and many sedentary men.

2,800: About right for teenage boys, many active men, and some very active women.

Servings from the:	1,600 cal.	2,200 cal.	2,800 cal.
Bread Group	6	9	11
Vegetable Group	3	4	5
Fruit Group	2	3	4
Milk Group	2-3*	2-3*	2-3*
Meat Group** (ounces)	5	6	7

*Women who are pregnant or breast-feeding, teenagers, and young adults to age 24 need 3 servings.
**Meat group amounts are in total ounces.

Building Blocks of Healthy Snacking

The Food Guide Pyramid depicts the importance of eating foods from a variety of food groups. Because every food offers different nutrients, eating a wide variety of foods helps you meet your nutrient needs. Avoid getting into a rut, eating the same snacks day after day. It all comes down to balancing your choices. You don't need to deny yourself foods that you enjoy; you simply need to find ways to incorporate them into your meals and snacks in sensible proportions.

Consider keeping a record of what you eat for several days and comparing it to the Food Guide Pyramid guidelines for varying calorie levels. On average, how does your diet rate? Do you need to eat more of certain food groups? Less of others? Consider how you can adjust these imbalances with your snack food choices. The nutrient information in Appendix A and guidelines in Appendix B can help you in selecting foods from each food group.

Mix and match snack foods. Turn your snacks into mini-meals by selecting foods from at least two of the food categories in the table below. For example, you might combine a mini-muffin from the grain group with yogurt from the milk, yogurt, cheese group. This combination approach helps to create snacks that make a meaningful contribution to your daily nutritional needs. Consider this, grains provide carbohydrates and B-vitamins. Fruits and vegetables offer vitamin A, vitamin C, carbohydrates, and fiber. Milk products are a good source of protein and calcium; when possible, though, try to select the lower fat versions of these foods. Meats, dried beans, eggs, and nuts are also good sources of protein, iron, and zinc, but some foods in this group also tend to be higher in fat, so look for lean and low-fat products or take smaller portions.

Mix-and-Match Snack Food Ideas

To build a mini-meal, select foods from at least two food categories.

Grain Group

❑ Bagel   ❑ Dry cereal

❑ Rice cakes   ❑ Low-fat snack crackers

❑ Low-fat graham crackers   ❑ Low-fat or mini-muffin

❑ Pita bread   ❑ Popcorn (unbuttered)

❑ Pretzels

Fruits & Vegetables

- ❏ Apple
- ❏ Canned fruit cup
- ❏ Celery sticks
- ❏ Grapes
- ❏ Kiwi fruit
- ❏ Peach or nectarine
- ❏ Banana
- ❏ Carrot sticks
- ❏ Dried fruit
- ❏ Green and red pepper strips
- ❏ Orange or tangerine
- ❏ Pear

Milk, Yogurt, & Cheese

- ❏ Cheese
- ❏ Frozen yogurt
- ❏ Nonfat or 1% milk
- ❏ Yogurt-based dip
- ❏ Cottage cheese
- ❏ Pudding
- ❏ Yogurt

Meats, Dried Beans, Eggs, & Nuts

- ❏ Ham
- ❏ Hard-boiled egg
- ❏ Leftover meat or poultry
- ❏ Peanut butter
- ❏ Turkey ham
- ❏ Hummus spread
- ❏ Lean luncheon meats
- ❏ Low-fat hot dogs
- ❏ Tuna
- ❏ Turkey hot dogs

Time your snacks. Another factor you'll want to consider as you choose your snacks is when you expect to eat next. The composition of your snack will determine how long you'll feel satisfied. Carbohydrate-containing foods (for example, breads, cereals, fruits, vegetables) are digested and absorbed fairly quickly, entering the bloodstream within 30 to 60 minutes. But fiber, found in whole grain foods and fruits and vegetables, tends to slow digestion and absorption. Foods that contain protein and fat (for example, milk, cheese, meats) make you feel full longer; they "stick to your ribs." This is because fat tends to slow the stomach's release of food into the intestines, and proteins take longer for the body to digest.

The size of the snack also will affect how long it takes to digest —more calories means a longer digestion time. A snack that contains a mixture of carbohydrate, fat, and protein will satisfy the immediate urge for food and keep hunger at bay for a longer time. If you need immediate, short-term satisfaction to hold off hunger for a short time, select snack foods containing primarily carbohydrates, such as grains, fruits, and vegetables.

A Lesson in Label Reading

Scanning food packages for nutrition information can help you select snacks that are the best nutritional bargains. Virtually all packaged foods now carry the distinctive Nutrition Facts label, and many products also feature claims about the nutritional content of the food.

Nutrient Claims

Food labeling regulations allow the terms low, light, and reduced to be paired with certain nutrients that most people need to eat in moderation: calories, fat, sodium, saturated fat, and cholesterol. Phrases like "high in..." and "good source of..." describe the levels of helpful nutrients, such as calcium, iron, fiber, vitamin C, and vitamin A. In order to make any of these claims, products must meet specific criteria, so you can trust that the claims are accurate. The following table defines some of the more common terms you'll see on food packages.

Deciphering Nutrient Claims

Claim	Criteria (per serving)	Comments
Low-calorie	40 calories or less	Note the serving size. If it's less than you usually eat, calories will be higher.
Reduced calorie	At least 25% less calories than a similar food	Depending on the calorie level of the similar food, the calories could still be high.
Light in calories	At least 1/3 fewer calories than a similar food	Depending on the calorie level of the similar food, the calories could still be high.
Fat-free	0.5 grams of fat or less	Usually means the lowest fat choice. Serving size may be less than what you'd typically eat.
Low-fat	3 grams of fat or less	If you only eat one serving, you can be assured of a low fat intake. But you still need to check the calories.
Reduced fat	At least 25% less fat than a similar food	If the full-fat cousin is extremely high in fat, the reduced fat food may still be quite high in fat.

Light in fat	At least 50% less fat than a similar food	Fat reduction is significant. Be sure to compare calorie level to the full-fat cousin.
High in	Contains 20% or more of the Daily Value	Used with dietary fiber, protein, vitamins, and minerals.
Good source of	Contains 10 to 19% of the Daily Value	Used with dietary fiber, protein, vitamins, and minerals.
More	Contains 10% more than a similar food	Used with dietary fiber, protein, vitamins, and minerals.

Nutrition Facts

Don't stop after reading the front of the package—this doesn't tell the whole story. Flip the package around until you find the Nutrition Facts panel. To guide your snack food choices, pay attention to the following:

Serving Size. Just below the "Nutrition Facts" title, you will find the serving size information. The serving size is listed in a user-friendly measure, such as 1 cup, 12 chips, 2 cookies. On packages that contain more than one serving, the number of servings per container also will be provided. Use the serving size information as a guide—if you eat more or less you'll need to adjust the nutrient information because it is based on the serving size stated. Be aware that the serving size on labels is not necessarily the recommended serving and may differ from serving sizes associated with the Food Guide Pyramid. Label serving sizes are based on amounts most commonly consumed.

Calories. Don't fall into the trap of thinking that low-fat, fat-free, or reduced fat means low calorie. Often when the fat level is reduced, more sugar and other ingredients, which boost the calorie level, are added to enhance the flavor. Also pay attention to portion sizes. You'll want to consider the serving size and nutrient content when choosing foods for snacks to determine if your choice is how you want to "spend" your calories. Keep in mind that foods high in calories and low in nutrients such as total carbohydrates, dietary fiber, vitamin A, vitamin C, iron, and calcium, are not the best nutritional bargains.

% Daily Values. The column to the right of the nutrients lists the percent Daily Value for each nutrient. The Daily Values listed on the bottom portion of the label represent the recommended amount of each nutrient you should eat in a day (based on a 2,000 calorie diet). The percentages show how much of these recommended amounts the food contributes to your overall intake. For example a % Daily Value for fat of 13% means that the product contains 13% of your daily need for fat. When choosing foods for snacks, look for high percentages of total carbohydrates, dietary fiber, vitamin A, vitamin C, iron, and calcium, and low percentages of fat, saturated fat, cholesterol, and sodium. Pair these facts with the calorie information. For instance, a product that is high-calorie and has 10% or more of the Daily Value for nutrients such as total carbohydrates, dietary fiber, vitamin A, vitamin C, iron, and calcium is a good calorie investment.

Nutrition Facts Panel

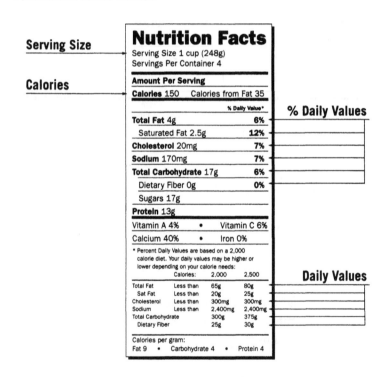

Myths (and Facts) About Snacking

Myth. Snacks spoil your appetite for meals.

Fact. Devouring a large snack just before a meal can spoil your appetite, but a small snack eaten 1 to 3 hours before a meal can actually keep you from becoming ravenously hungry and prevent you from overeating.

Myth. Snacking causes cavities.

Fact. Frequent snacking doesn't cause cavities, but it can promote them. The longer teeth come in contact with food, particularly carbohydrate foods, the more time bacteria in plaque has to produce acids that damage tooth enamel.

Myth. Snacking causes weight gain.

Fact. It depends on how you snack. Regular snacking on large amounts of high-calorie foods can cause weight gain, but well-timed, nutritious snacks can actually help to control your weight. Eating a snack that makes a nutritional contribution to your diet during the long stretches between meals can take the edge off hunger and prevent overeating

Myth. Snacking is a bad habit.

Fact. As long as your snacking habits follow the food choice guidelines outlined by the Food Guide Pyramid, you can build a balanced diet that includes snacks. Snacking can be a problem if you frequently splurge on the foods at the top of the Pyramid, eating them in addition to, or instead of, other more nutrient-rich foods.

Myth. Children should be taught not to snack.

Fact. Actually, children need snacks. Children have high energy needs and small stomachs. They're not able to eat enough food in just three meals to get all the nutrients and calories they need. That's why children should be taught healthy snacking habits.

Myth. Snack foods labeled low-fat are also low in calories.

Fact. When comparing the Nutrition Facts panel of a low-fat or fat-free food to its full-fat counterpart, you'll see that the calories from fat will be lower, but be sure to compare the total calories and the size of the serving this information is based on. Many foods that are reformulated to reduce the fat content have other ingredients, such as sugar, added to improve the flavor. These ingredients may boost the total calories to be as high as, or even higher than,

Building Blocks of Healthy Snacking

their full-fat counterparts. If you're watching your fat intake, these products can be helpful, but depending on the food and the type of claim (low-fat vs. reduced fat vs. fat-free), the fat savings may not be tremendous. Also keep in mind that consuming more calories than your body needs over time results in excess body fat and weight gain. The bottom line is: pay attention to calories and fat, watch your portion sizes, and don't let low-fat lure you into thinking it's calorie-free.

Myth. Sugar is bad for your health.

Fact. A potential problem with sugary foods is that they can take the place of other, more nutritious foods in your diet. For children, this can create serious problems over time, such as becoming overweight. Frequent sugar consumption also promotes tooth decay. But sugar alone does not cause diabetes, hyperactivity, or any other serious health problems. A modest amount of sugar and sweet foods, balanced with other more nutritious foods, has a place in the diet.

Chapter Two

Snacking
and Children

MANY PARENTS STILL HANG ON to the outdated view that snacking is a bad habit, and they limit their children's between-meal eating. We now know that children actually need to snack. As a parent, you should know how snacking fits into your child's eating pattern—when and where to offer snacks, what to serve, and how much. You'll also discover that getting children involved in preparing snacks makes them more interested and enthused about all the food you serve. A healthy and fun approach to snacking during infancy and childhood helps to lay the groundwork for a lifetime of healthy snacking.

Why Kids Need Snacks

Children's energy needs are high for two simple reasons: they're growing and they're usually quite active. In fact, even though children's bodies are smaller than adults, their total energy needs are comparable to adults. Moreover, children actually need more calories per pound of body weight than adults. From 1 to 3 years of age, the recommended calorie intake for a child weighing 29 pounds is 1,300 (ranging from 900 to 1,800). From 4 to 6 years of age, the calorie requirement for a 44-pound child is 1,700 (ranging from 1,300 to 2,300). From 7 to 10 years of age, the average calorie requirement (2,400) exceeds that of most adult women. Despite high energy needs, children's stomachs have a small capacity for food. They get full after eating a small amount. That's why children need to eat every 3 or 4 hours throughout the day to meet their total calorie needs and maintain a steady supply of energy.

Lifelong eating habits are formed during childhood, so this is the time to instill a balanced approach to snacking. If snacks are treated like a "forbidden fruit," curiosity and temptation can cause kids to overdo it when they get a chance. On the other hand, exposing children to a variety of nutritious snacks and building snacking into their eating patterns shows them how to fit snacks into a balanced diet.

The Scoop on Sugar

As a parent, you may have concerns about serving your child sugary snacks. Besides enhancing flavor and acceptability, sugar actually serves a variety of important functions in food—it helps food retain moisture, prevents spoilage, and improves texture and appearance. Because sugar alone provides calories but no vitamins or minerals, it is considered an empty-calorie food. Over time, eating a lot of empty calories, in addition to other foods, can cause a child to gain weight. Still, children's energy needs are high enough that they can handle some empty calories, especially if your child is active.

Problems occur when sugary foods take the place of more nutritious foods in the diet, depriving your child of important nutrients. For example, regularly substituting soft drinks for milk can result in a shortage of calcium. And sugar, especially sugary foods that dissolve slowly in your mouth or stick to your teeth (like hard candy, chewing gum, raisins), contribute to tooth decay. Despite popular beliefs, sugar does not cause diabetes, hyperactivity, or any other significant health problems.

Given these facts, you probably don't want to make high-sugar, low-nutrient foods (such as soft drinks and candy) a staple of your child's diet, but you don't need to ban them either. Complete restriction can even backfire. Some children raised in sugar-free households load up on sweets when they're away from home. The best approach is to offer sweets occasionally, combining them with other nutrient-dense foods (for example, cookies with milk).

A Game Plan for Snacking

Randomly selected snacks eaten any time of the day can lead to a number of nutrition problems (for example, excess calorie intake, weight gain, inability to distinguish hunger and fullness or satiety, inadequate nutrient intake). For young children, it's important for an adult to oversee when snacks are served and the type of food served. The way to regulate snacking is to be ahead of the game—select reasonable times for snacks and put food on the table, just as you would serve a meal. As children get older, your best strategy is to have plenty of healthy snacks on hand and to teach them how to make healthy choices.

When. Snacks should be offered at consistent times of the day. Ideally, serve snacks midway between meals—long enough after a meal so your child learns to eat enough to feel satisfied and at least 1 to 2 hours before the next meal. Postponing snacks until a few hours after a meal will help prevent a child from refusing the food served at a meal and then immediately begging for food. This pattern of very small feedings throughout the day can actually result in insufficient calorie and nutrient intake in young children. Furthermore, few parents are interested in being a short-order cook! On the other hand, snacking immediately before a meal can dull the appetite. Serve snacks early enough so that your child will be hungry and look forward to mealtime.

In some households, it may be necessary to serve two snacks if there is a long interval between meals. Case in point: let's look at 3-year old Jennifer whose working parents typically serve dinner between 7:00 and 8:00 p.m. Because her child care center serves lunch at 11:30 a.m. and afternoon snack at 3:00 p.m., Jennifer was famished at 5:30 p.m. when her father picked her up, and she fussed inconsolably during the 45-minute commute home. Her parents realized that they needed to arrange for Jennifer to have a larger mid-afternoon snack that contained protein, carbohydrate, and fat (for example, peanut butter or cheese on crackers or rice cakes, or bagels and cream cheese with milk) at the day care center. Then dad served Jennifer a light, carbohydrate snack she could eat during the ride home. He offered fruit, vegetables, pretzels, cereal, or rice cakes which took the edge off Jennifer's hunger without spoiling her appetite for dinner. This approach met Jennifer's nutrient needs and resulted in a more peaceful ride home.

Where. When at home, limit snacking to certain locations, such as the kitchen and dining room. This helps to keep snacking a structured and purposeful eating experience. Many unconscious patterns of overeating stem from eating all over the house and while engaged in other activities. Adhering to designated eating locations also reduces spills on floors and furniture!

With the active pace of today's lifestyles there are bound to be snack times when you're in the car or out and about. In these situations, the time of the snack is more important than the location. It's not a good idea to wait until a child is famished before offering a snack. If possible, take a break where you can find a table to eat. But realize that you also need to be flexible and adaptable. In reality, we're a nation of people who eat on the run and in unusual places.

What. When selecting foods for snacks, keep the Food Guide Pyramid (page 5) in mind. First, consider what your child typically eats during meals, and then fill in the gaps with snacks. You may want to write down what your child eats for a few days, comparing his or her intake to the Food Guide Pyramid. If your child's intake typically falls short of the recommended servings from a specific food group, add these foods in the form of snacks. Some traditional snack foods, like candy, belong in the tip of the Pyramid (fats, oils, and sweets) and should be eaten sparingly. Although watching fats and sweets is prudent, children have special dietary needs which influence the recommendations for fat and sugar. Within each food group, go easy on foods that are high in sodium or salt, especially for infants and toddlers whose immature kidneys have a hard time clearing excess sodium.

Also keep in mind that the composition and size of your child's snacks will help determine how long hunger will kept at bay. More calories means longer digestion time. And, serving snacks that contain a mixture of carbohydrate, fat, and protein will satisfy a child's hunger for a longer time than a snack containing primarily carbohydrate, such as crackers, pretzels, or fruit. On the other hand, when snacks are served shortly before a meal to take the edge off hunger, it's better to offer primarily carbohydrate-containing foods.

Like adults, children may grow tired of the same foods day after day, so try to vary the snacks you serve. Eating a wide variety of foods is also a key nutrition strategy, because every food offers different nutrients. For example, incorporate seasonal fruits and vegetables into your child's snacks. You'll be able to take advantage of produce at its best while varying what you serve—apples in the fall, oranges in the winter, strawberries in early summer, and peaches, pears, and cantaloupe in the late summer. Grapes, kiwi, and bananas are available all year to intersperse with these seasonal offerings. And don't forget about canned and frozen fruit, which also introduce more variety and don't spoil. Different flavors of fruit juice, yogurt, and pudding spice up routine snacks. A variety of dry cereals, cracker and pretzel shapes, and dried fruit can be combined in different ways to make trail mix snacks.

Do Young Children Need Fat?

Well-meaning parents have heeded the general warnings about fat, adopting a low-fat diet for their children, as well as themselves. But guidelines that promote a decrease in the amount of fat we eat do not apply to young children (age 5 and younger). In fact, severe fat restriction in young children can cause impaired growth and development. Because their energy needs are so high, including fat in a child's diet is important. Fat is a concentrated source of calories. It contains more than twice as many calories per gram (9 calories/gram) as compared to carbohydrate and protein (4 calories/gram). In contrast to adults, who should limit fat to no more than 30 percent of total calories, young children need approximately 30 to 40 percent of their calories from fat to support growth and development. For a child consuming 1,800 calories per day, this translates to about 60 to 80 grams of fat per day.

After 2 years of age, children should gradually adopt a diet that, by about 5 years of age, contains no more than 30 percent of calories from fat. The bottom line is that you don't need to be as concerned about selecting low-fat foods for children as you do for yourself.

How Much. Snacks should supplement, not replace, meals for children, and portions should be child-size. As a rule of thumb, serve one-fourth to one-third of an adult portion or 1 tablespoon for every year of life. Children can become overwhelmed with adult-size portions, sometimes eating less than they otherwise would. It's always better to give less than you think your child will eat, then offer seconds if your child is still hungry and it's not too close to mealtime.

Allow your child to control the amount of food eaten. Children are born with the ability to signal when they are full, but parents sometimes miss the cues. Newborns stop sucking, play with the nipple, and turn their heads away; one year olds shake their heads and push unwanted food aside. Trust your instincts on this matter; a child who is forced to keep eating when full may lose touch with his or her internal signals of hunger and fullness. Toddlers, even though they are able to say they are full, can be a little more difficult to read because they are so easily distracted and may want to return to their play. If you suspect that your child is more distracted than full, gently bring the focus back to eating, but don't force the issue. Children's appetites fluctuate, but they usually find a reasonable balance over time.

Preparing Snacks—Get Kids Involved

Children not only enjoy being involved in food preparation and selection but they often show more interest in eating foods they've helped to select and prepare. You may even want to designate a shelf or area of the refrigerator for children's snacks, allowing them to select their own foods from this section.

There are many steps of food preparation children can assist. For example, two- and three-year-olds can peel bananas, tear lettuce, place bread in a toaster, and arrange slices of food. Four- and five-year-olds can cut soft foods with a table knife, spread toppings, make simple sandwiches, pour liquids, and assist with measuring ingredients.

Kids in the Kitchen

All these activities require adult supervision.

Two and Three Year Olds Can:

➤ Wash hands

➤ Wash fruits and vegetables

➤ Place paper liners in muffin tins

➤ Tear lettuce

➤ Peel bananas

- ➤ Throw waste in trash can
- ➤ Place unbreakable dishes on the table
- ➤ Help count the proper number of spoonfuls or cupfuls

Four and Five Year Olds Can Also:
- ➤ Pour broken eggs from bowl into mixture
- ➤ Open packages and pour into bowl
- ➤ Mix dry and wet ingredients
- ➤ Knead and shape dough
- ➤ Make simple sandwiches
- ➤ Pour cereal and dry ingredients
- ➤ Set the table
- ➤ Handle a table knife (cutting and spreading)

Six Year Olds and Older Can Also:
- ➤ Break eggs into a bowl
- ➤ Stir hot liquids
- ➤ Gather ingredients from cupboards and refrigerator
- ➤ Pour liquids
- ➤ Measure ingredients
- ➤ Pour liquids with assistance

Simple snacks that require minimal preparation are practical on a day-to-day basis, but remember that children get excited about foods that are fun and interesting. Fortunately, with a number of simple techniques, you can make foods more enticing for children. Here are a few ideas:

Jazz up fruits and vegetables with peanut butter. Let kids decorate apple slices, celery sticks, cucumber slices, and carrot sticks with peanut butter and raisins.

Cut food into various shapes. Quarter sandwiches into small triangles or squares, or create "sandwich fingers" by cutting a sandwich into five long slices.

Allow your child to pick the shape of their snack. Offer cheese cubes or cheese slices, pizza squares or triangles.

Use cookie cutters to make an assortment of shapes from bread. Then let your child add the toppings (use the edges to make croutons or bread crumbs). Older kids can spread cream cheese, peanut butter, or cheese spread. Younger kids can decorate with sliced, chopped, and grated vegetables: green and red pepper strips, olives slices, celery slices or sticks, cucumber slices, and grated or sliced carrots.

Safety and Cleanliness

Don't forget about safety and cleanliness when letting your child help with food preparation. Washing hands before handling food or equipment is a good habit to instill; children's hands come in contact with a lot of dirt and germs through their play. Teach them to use a clean spoon for tasting. Keep handles of pots and pans turned away from the front of the stove. Insist that your child stands back when you are using power equipment to chop, slice, blend, or mix food. Warn them when hot grease may spatter, and make them stand clear of a hot oven. Do not leave young children alone in the kitchen while preparing food.

Snacking On the Go

Today's busy parents benefit from numerous advances in packaging which cater to younger consumers and require little or no food preparation. A wide range of healthy snacks come ready-to-eat out of the container—and children love these packages because they're the right size and often graphically appealing. Juice boxes, single serve boxes of animal crackers, cheese sticks, single-serve puddings and applesauce, and mini rice cakes can be thrown into a backpack, diaper bag, or picnic basket for snacking on the run. Although these products also make snack time at home very convenient and satisfying, they tend to be more expensive. You can create your own single-servings by dividing the contents of larger packages into small, reusable storage containers or snack-size zipper storage bags.

Smart Snacks for Infants and Toddlers

Once a baby can sit upright in a high chair and use her thumb and forefinger (the pincer grip) to pick up foods, finger foods can be incorporated into the diet. When selecting snack foods for older infants and toddlers up to 3 and 4 years of age, be aware of potential choking hazards. Never leave babies and toddlers unsupervised while eating, especially when trying new foods.

Choking Hazards for Children Under 3-4 Years

Small, Hard Foods	Slippery Foods
Nuts	Whole grapes
Seeds	Large pieces of meats and poultry
Popcorn	Frankfurters
Snack chips	Candy
Pretzels	Cough drops
Raw carrots	Chewing gum
Snack puffs	Raisins

Introducing snacks into your baby's eating routine at 8 to 10 months helps the transition to table foods. Small pieces of dry cereal, such as O-shaped cereal, stimulate a baby's pincer grip, as well as hand-to-mouth coordination. Soft foods (for example, pieces of bread, bananas, pears, peaches, or kiwifruit) cut into small pieces (1/2" to 1" chunks) encourage chewing. Milk or juice from a sippy cup or straw cup served with snacks help the transition from the bottle or breast at about one year of age. Gradually replacing morning and afternoon bottle- or breast-feedings with snack foods helps your baby learn that eating is a sitting-up affair that involves food, not just milk.

Some parents, afraid to serve table foods until teeth have appeared, wait too long to start finger foods and their baby becomes dependent on spoon feeding. Although choking is a real concern, serving soft finger foods will stimulate oral development and aid the transition to table foods. The first teeth in the front are used for biting, and the molars (which are not all in place until a baby is around 2 years old) grind food. Before the molars arrive, babies can gum soft food to a smooth consistency; this gumming process stimulates chewing skills. Canned fruits and vegetables are the perfect texture for promoting gumming skills. Canned vegetables can be high in sodium—buy the reduced-sodium products or rinse them before serving. You can also prepare soft finger foods by cooking raw fruits and fresh or frozen vegetables in the microwave for a few minutes (for example, peeled and diced apples, carrots, potatoes, or peas). Once a baby has front teeth and learns to bite off reasonably sized pieces of food, you can offer larger pieces of food, such as sandwiches cut in quarters, cheese sticks or slices, mini-muffins, and slices of bread. There will be a mess, but these larger pieces of food teach self-feeding skills.

After your child's 2-year molars are in and chewing skills are mastered, a wider range of foods can be served. You can offer larger pieces and serve fruits and vegetables with skins (for example, apples, grapes, nectarines, plums). When introducing these foods, you should still take precautions for choking until you are certain that your child can safely handle these foods.

The following tables offer snack food and mini-meal ideas for young children according to age. The age at which your child can manage the foods listed may vary. You are the best judge of when your child is ready to progress.

Snack Foods for Older Infants, Toddlers, and Pre-schoolers

When introducing new foods, watch for signs of a food allergy or intolerance. Signs include a skin rash, wheezing, diarrhea, or vomiting. Foods that may cause a reaction include egg white, citrus fruits, cow's milk, and peanut butter. It is best to hold off introducing these foods until after 1 year of age, then introduce them one at a time and monitor for a reaction. Foods containing wheat can also cause a reaction. Introduce rice, barley, and oatmeal cereals before wheat .

Grains

8 Months to 2 Years	3 and 4 Years
Animal crackers	Animal crackers
Bread and rolls	Bagels
Bread sticks	Bread and rolls
Dry cereal, unsweetened, small pieces	Bread sticks
	Cinnamon or raisin toast
Graham crackers	Corn bread
Muffins	Dry cereal, unsweetened
Pancakes	English muffins
Rice cakes	Graham crackers
Teething biscuits	Muffins
Waffles	Pancakes
	Pretzels
	Rice cakes
	Snack crackers
	Popcorn
	Tortillas
	Waffles

Fruit

8 Months to 2 Years

Apples, diced and cooked
Applesauce
Banana, sliced and quartered
Cantaloupe
Kiwi fruit, peeled and cubed
Honeydew melon
Peaches, cut fresh or canned
Pears, cut fresh or canned

3 and 4 Years

Apple slices, raw
Applesauce
Banana, whole or half
Cantaloupe
Dried fruit
Grapes, seedless
Kiwi fruit, peeled and sliced
Honeydew melon
Orange slices
Peaches
Pears
Pineapple
Raisins
Strawberries
Tangerines

Vegetables

Broccoli, cut and cooked
Cauliflower, cut and cooked
Carrots, sliced and cooked
Green beans, canned or cooked
Peas, canned or frozen and thawed
Potato, cooked and cubed
  or mashed
Sweet potato, cooked and
  cubed or mashed

Broccoli, cooked or raw
Cauliflower, cooked or raw
Carrots, cooked or raw
Celery sticks
Cucumber slices
Green beans, canned
  or cooked
Green and red pepper slices
Peas, canned or frozen
  and thawed
Squash, cubed and cooked

Milk, Yogurt, Cheese

Formula or breast milk until 1 year
  Whole milk after 1 year
Cheese, cubes or slices
Cheese sticks
Cottage cheese
Frozen yogurt
Pudding, whole milk
Yogurt, whole milk

1% or 2% after 2 years
Cheese, cubes or slices
Cheese sticks
Cottage cheese
Frozen yogurt
Pudding
Yogurt

Snacking and Children

23

Meat, Poultry, Fish, Eggs, Dry Beans and Nuts

8 Months to 2 Years

Leftover meats, cut in 1/2" pieces
Peanut butter on crackers or bread
Refried beans rolled in tortilla
   and sliced
Hard cooked eggs
   (no egg whites before
   1 year of age)

3 and 4 Years

Hotdogs or turkey dogs
Leftover meats
Luncheon meats
Peanut butter on crackers,
   bread, or fruit
Refried beans rolled in tortilla
   . and sliced
Tuna
Hard cooked eggs

For nutrition information, refer to Appendix A.

Mini-Meals for Older Infants and Toddlers

8 Months to 2 Years

Animal crackers (10)

Apple, cooked pieces (1/4 cup)

Milk, whole (1/2 c.)

> **Calories 200**
> **Fat 7g**

Graham crackers (2 squares)

Peanut butter (2 tsp.)

Milk, whole (1/2 c.)

Banana (1/4)

> **Calories 285**
> **Fat 13g**

Cheerios (1/4 cup)

Cheese stick (1)

Kiwi fruit (1/2)

Apple juice (1/2 cup)

> **Calories 175**
> **Fat 5g**

Cooked carrot slices (1/4 cup)

Bread sticks (2)

Milk, whole (1/2 c.)

> **Calories 175**
> **Fat 6g**

Pancake (1) spread with peanut butter (2 tsp.)

Vanilla pudding (1/2 cup)

Milk, whole (1/2 c.)

Calories 265
Fat 12g

2 to 3 Years

Cottage cheese and peaches, blended (1/4 cup)

Whole wheat crackers (10 bite size)

Apple juice (3/4 c.)

Calories 250
Fat 7g

Apple slices, peeled (1/2 cup)

Peanut butter (1 Tbsp.)

Raisins (2 Tbsp.)

Graham crackers (2 whole)

Calories 300
Fat 12g

Trail mix (dry cereal, raisins, pretzels) (1 cup)

Baby carrots (3)

Wild cherry juice (1/2 c.)

Calories 180
Fat 1g

Pear (1/2)

Brick cheese (1 oz.)

Whole wheat crackers (10 bite-size)

White grape juice (1/2 c.)

Calories 330
Fat 14g

Cottage cheese (1/4 cup) mixed with applesauce (1/4 c.),
    cinnamon, and raisins (2 Tbsp.)

Graham crackers (2 whole)

Apple juice (1/2 c.)

Calories 310
Fat 5g

Smart Snacks for Older Kids

By the time children are 4 years old, they have mastered feeding themselves and can safely eat most foods. Your child should also start to play a bigger role in selecting and preparing food. If you've laid the groundwork for healthy snacking, this process of gradually transferring responsibility to your child can be enjoyable. Your school-age child will likely want to control snack selection and preparation. You can help by stocking your pantry and refrigerator with the makings of healthy snacks and helping your child combine snack foods into mini-meals that build a balanced diet. However, if your child has developed food-related problem behaviors (such as refusing entire food groups or eating very few foods), you'll want to remain more involved in the selection and preparation of snacks.

Mini-Meals for Older Kids (4+ Years)

Fruit kabobs (pineapple, cantaloupe, bananas, grapes skewered on toothpicks) (1/2 cup fruit)

Cheese sticks (1)

Mini-bagel (1)

Calories 215
Fat 5g

Bean burrito with cheese (1)

Applesauce (1/2 cup)

Mineral water

Calories 240
Fat 6g

Raisin toast (2 slices) with butter or margarine (2 tsp.)

Fruit yogurt, low-fat (1 cup)

Cantaloupe melon cubes (1 cup)

Calories 375
Fat 8g

Trail mix (dry cereal, raisins, pretzels, nuts) (1 cup)

Carrot and celery sticks (4)

Wild cherry juice (1/2 c.)

Calories 355
Fat 10g

Banana (1/2) dipped in orange juice (1 Tbsp.) and rolled in granola
(1 Tbsp.)

Oatmeal cookie (1)

Milk, 1% (1 cup)

Calories 205
Fat 5g

Tortilla chips (20)

Green and red pepper slices (1/2 cup)

Mild salsa (2 Tbsp.)

Mineral water

Calories 140
Fat 6g

Smoothie—puree in a blender:

—orange juice (1/2 cup)

—strawberries (2-3 whole)

—banana (1/2)

—yogurt, plain nonfat (1/4 cup)

Calories 155
Fat 1g

Chapter Three

Snacking and Teens

SNACKS AND TEENAGERS seem to go hand in hand. The fact is, teenagers' lifestyles are conducive to snacking. Schedules are often packed and erratic. School, part-time jobs, athletics, social activities, and extra-curricular programs make regular meals difficult. And skipped meals are common, particularly breakfast and dinner.

Healthful snacks, or mini-meals, can fill nutritional gaps and accommodate teenagers' active lifestyles. For example, a carton of yogurt with a raisin bagel is a reasonable substitute for breakfast, and it provides calcium, protein, and iron. Portable snacks—dried fruit, power bars, trail mix, bagels, cheese sticks, pretzels, and fruit—provide fuel for after-school athletic practices and competitions. For many teens, especially those involved in sports, snacking is the only way to meet high nutritional needs in a time-crunched lifestyle. For many teenagers, snacks make up 25 to 33 percent of an average day's calorie intake.

Why Teens Need Healthy Snacks

Snacks make sense for anyone who is busy, but there are physical reasons why teenagers need snacks. Calorie and nutrient needs soar because of rapid growth during the teenage years, which rival infancy in terms of dramatic physical changes. Although there is a wide individual variation, girls typically experience a growth spurt between the ages of 10 and 13; boys between the ages of 12 and 15 years. During this period of rapid growth, girls grow about 10 inches and gain approximately 35 pounds. They also become calorie-conscious, often pursuing drastic measures to control their weight. Boys, on the other hand, grow about 12 inches and gain approximately 45 pounds.

Teenagers' calorie and nutrient needs are higher than at any other time of life, with the exception of pregnancy and breast-feeding. For the average teen girl, the recommended calorie intake is about 2,200 per day, and for the average teen boy it's about 3,000. But calorie needs vary tremendously. A small, 15-year-old girl whose growth is complete may need 1,800 calories or less; an active boy of the same age, at the peak of his growth, could need 4,000 calories a day. These high calorie needs can be hard to meet with three meals a day, so snacks can make important calorie and nutrient contributions to intense teenage growth demands.

Not any snack will do, however. A number of nutrition problems arise when meals are replaced with empty-calorie snacks such as chips, French fries, soft drinks, candy bars, pastries, and cookies. For example, swapping soft drinks for milk can compromise calcium intake, weakening bones and increasing the risk of osteoporosis later in life. Eating a lot of high-fat and high-cholesterol snacks lays the groundwork for heart disease—for both boys and girls. For many teenage girls, skipped meals seem to be a way to curb calorie intake, but this approach often leads to binge eating on high-fat snacks, and consequently, excess calorie intake.

Food, Friends, and Freedom

Teenagers are striking out on their own, making many more choices than they did as children. Yet at the same time, a variety of social and emotional issues influence their choices: peer acceptance, searching for their identity, mistrust of authority, and struggling for independence. The teenage years represent a time of intense emotional highs and lows, a process of self-discovery, and a period of change and uncertainty. Food choices and eating habits, like all other aspects of their lives, are affected by these dynamics.

Peer Pressure. School cafeterias, fast food restaurants, convenience stores, pizza parlors, and malls are social gathering grounds for teenagers. Many teenagers find it awkward, and even humiliating, to make food choices that deviate from their friends' selections, even if they prefer different foods. They may find it easier to follow the crowd, eating what everyone else is eating. Quite often, the group is ordering burgers, fries, chips, and soft drinks.

Struggle for Independence. As many parents of teenagers are made to feel—no one knows less about anything than a parent. Resisting authority figures is a natural part of fighting for independence. This can make it hard for parents to offer nutritional guidance, especially if they are undergoing a power struggle with their child. Teenagers may not only think that their parents are wrong, but so are home economics and health teachers, doctors, nurses, government authorities, and other experts. Coaches may be able to influence teenage athletes, but a coach's ability to provide nutritional guidance often is limited. Imparting accurate nutritional information and guidance to teenagers in a way that it is heard and valued can be a challenge.

Invincible to Future Ills. For many teenagers, the future is far away— some nebulous unknown with little meaning. They feel invincible— immune to chronic diseases, such as cancer and heart disease, that strike adults. Teenagers sometimes have a hard time seeing and accepting how choices they make today will affect them later; if they understand this relationship, they may not care. Nutritional advice needs to relate to what matters to teenagers today.

· ·

For Parents Only

As a parent, your role as gatekeeper of nutritional information and food choices for your teenager is diminishing. If you laid the groundwork during childhood, instilling good eating habits at an early age, you've done what you can. At this point, you can continue to be a good role model and keep your pantry and refrigerator stocked with nutritious snacks. If your teenager turns to you for help in solving nutritional problems and concerns (for example, how to get enough to eat when classes last all day and practice begins right after school), you can serve as a sounding board, helping your child find practical solutions. You also can support the follow-through (for example, buying and packing portable snacks).

· ·

A Snacking Reality Check

Teenagers, not unlike many others, typically care most about their personal interests—maybe it's sports or music or just hanging out with friends. To help teenagers improve their food choices, explain that eating every three to four hours fuels the brain and nerves, helping him stay alert and active so he has the energy to do the things he enjoys. Teenage bodies need more than empty calories (something to squelch hunger); they need vitamins and minerals to grow and develop and to fight infections. Healthy snacks can do both jobs.

What Motivates Girls? Girls tend to be most concerned with their appearance—clear skin, beautiful hair, and a slim figure. When discussing food and nutrition, talk to girls about how good nutrition creates beauty from the inside out—a healthy glow from head to foot. Selecting nutrient-dense foods (low calorie foods that are packed with vitamins and minerals) will help a teenage girl control her weight without depriving her of needed nutrients. (Refer to Chapter 5, Snacking for the Weight Conscious, for more information.)

. . . .

For Girls Only

Eating well can enhance your beauty from the inside out—giving you a healthy glow that make-up and clothing cannot provide. Healthy skin and hair need nutrients found in wholesome foods.

A healthy diet also makes you feel more energetic and lively. Your need for iron is high because iron in your blood is lost each month during your period. If you don't eat enough iron-rich foods to replace this lost iron, you may develop iron-deficiency anemia. Anemia makes you very tired and weak. Meats (such as hamburgers, steaks, chicken) are the best sources of iron, but snacking on raisins and enriched grain products (for example, cereal, bread, bagels, English muffins) also can help to boost your iron intake.

Regular meals and snacks of healthy foods give you a steady supply of energy. When you go for more than four hours without eating, your brain and nervous system do not have the fuel they need to function. This leaves you feeling tired and crabby, making it hard to concentrate and cope with stress. Going for long stretches without food also makes your body crave food. Believe it or not, the best way to control your weight is to eat three to five times a day. When choosing snack foods, look for foods that are low in calories but packed with nutrients (see the food lists in Chapter 5, Snacking for the Weight Conscious).

. . . .

What Motivates Boys? Boys are more likely to care more about their physique, striving for a tall stature, bulky muscles, and athletic prowess. Although genetics are the major determinants of stature and body build, good nutrition and exercise can help a teenage boy achieve his potential. Explain that to build muscles, they need extra exercise and extra calories. But the right kind of calories are important—more carbohydrate, moderate protein, and less fat. Fruits, vegetables, grains, and low-fat dairy products are great snacking choices for teenage boys who seek power, strength, and speed.

For Guys Only

Healthy snacks can provide the extra calories your body needs to grow taller and stronger. Loading up on fried chicken, greasy burgers, fries, and chips may satisfy your hunger, but these foods alone do not provide the right balance of nutrients. To build muscle, you need to combine weight-bearing exercise with meals and snacks consisting of mostly carbohydrates, some fat, and a moderate amount of protein. Eating lean meats, fish, or poultry twice a day will provide the protein you need to build muscles. Snacking on fruits, vegetables, grains, and low-fat dairy products will help to fuel your muscles for power, strength, and speed.

Healthy snacks also help to prevent energy slumps. Going for more than four hours without eating deprives your brain, nerves, and muscles of the fuel needed to function. This leaves you feeling sluggish and weak, making it hard to concentrate and perform.

Special Needs of Teenage Athletes

For teenagers involved in sports and athletics, fitting nutritious meals and snacks into a jam-packed schedule can be particularly challenging. Teen athletes need more calories to meet their high-energy needs; this means more food, whether from eating larger portions and/or eating more often. But between school, training, practices, and competitions, it can be hard to find time to eat. Athletes not only need more energy, they also need a specific type of fuel (see Chapter 4, Snacking for Fitness and Athletic Performance, for more information). Carbohydrates are the body's favorite fuel, and most types of exercise rely on carbohydrates to supply energy to the muscles. Without enough carbohydrates, an athlete will not have the stamina for peak performance.

The most important nutrient for active people is water. On a hot day, an athlete exercising hard for an hour can lose 3 quarts of water. During exercise, thirst sensations do not keep pace with fluid losses. So, by the time you feel thirsty, you're already dehydrated. To prevent dehydration, teenagers should drink:

➤ 8 to 24 fluid ounces of liquids an hour before exercise
➤ another 4 to 6 fluid ounces 5 to 20 minutes before exercise
➤ 4 to 6 fluid ounces every 15 to 20 minutes during exercise

Water, juice, or sports drinks are all fine choices. The carbonation in soft drinks can causing bloating and discomfort during exercise. In addition, the sugar concentration is too high, so fluids are not absorbed as quickly.

Aside from water and carbohydrates, athletes need a balanced diet to obtain essential nutrients. Refer to the Food Guide Pyramid (page 5) for guidance on how to build a balanced diet. Foods at the base of the Pyramid—grains, fruits, and vegetables—are the carbohydrate choices. Aim for the maximum number of servings of these foods.

But how can a teenager fit all this eating into a busy schedule? Portable snacks are one solution. Stashing snacks that won't spoil— granola bars, fruit bars, rice cakes, low-fat cookies and crackers, low-fat trail mix, dried fruit, mineral water, juice boxes, sports drinks—in lockers and gym bags is another solution. Fruit, bagels, yogurt, pudding, and other perishable foods can be carried in an insulated lunch sack with a cold pack for eating throughout the day.

Smart Snacks for Teens

Because teens tend to consume fewer carbohydrates and less calcium and iron than is recommended, snacks are a perfect opportunity to make up for these shortfalls. Dairy products provide calcium, so aim for three servings a day. Select the fat-free, reduced fat, or low-fat versions of milk, yogurt, pudding, cottage cheese, cheese spreads, and hard cheeses; many of these products taste as good as their full-fat cousins. Enriched breads and cereals from the grain group supply carbohydrates, as well as iron. Mini-bagels, rice cakes, pretzels, and low-fat crackers and cookies are easy to eat on the run. Refer to Appendix A for a list of snack foods and their nutrient contributions and Appendix B for guidance on selecting snacks.

> Mix and match foods from different food groups to turn snacks into mini-meals—experiment with different combinations. (Refer to the table "Mini-Meals for Teens" below for ideas for how to combine snack foods.) For example, pair a grain food with a dairy food; low-fat cookies with nonfat milk or pudding, fat-free cream cheese on a mini-bagel, and reduced fat cheese with low-fat snack crackers are tasty and fast.

> Snacks can be leftovers—eaten hot or cold.

> A microwave can be a snacker's best friend. At home, microwave a potato and add toppings.

> Make mini-pizzas from bagels or English muffins in the toaster oven or broiler.

> Blend cottage cheese or fat-free cream cheese with low-fat yogurt or sour cream to make vegetable dips and toppings/spreads for baked potatoes or sandwiches. Use different breads—pita pockets, raisin bread, foccacia, bagels, potato bread—for sandwiches to break the monotony of an old standby.

> Toss fruit, yogurt, fruit juice, and ice cubes into a blender to make a smoothie.

Mini-Meals for Teens

Pizza bagel (2 whole wheat bagel halves spread with 3 Tbsp. tomato paste or pizza sauce, sprinkled with 4 Tbsp. grated mozzarella cheese)

Carrot sticks (1 whole)

Diet soft drink, juice, or water
Calories 280
Fat 6g

Reduced fat chocolate sandwich cookies (2)

Nonfat milk (1 cup)

Apple (1 medium)
Calories 275
Fat 3g

Fat-free wheat snack crackers (1 oz.)
Herbed cottage cheese (1%) dip (1/4 cup)
Carrot (1/2 whole) and celery (1/2 stalk) sticks
Mineral water
> **Calories 150**
> **Fat 0.5g**

Trail mix (dry cereal, raisins, pretzels) (1 cup)
Low-fat fruit yogurt (1 cup)
Apple-raspberry juice (1 1/2 c.)
> **Calories 525**
> **Fat 4g**

Baked potato (cooked in microwave for 10 minutes). Add your
  choice of toppings and cook 2 -3 minutes more:
  —cottage cheese (1%) (1/4 cup)
  —fat-free sour cream or yogurt (1/4 cup)
  —cheddar cheese (2 oz.)
Raw cauliflower (1/2 cup) and baby carrots (3)
Ice water
> **Calories 200**
> **Fat 1g**
> Nutrient analysis based on cottage cheese

Tortilla chips, low-fat (20)
Green and red pepper slices (1/2 cup)
Salsa (1/4 cup)
Mineral water
> **Calories 175**
> **Fat 5g**

Raisin bagel (1) with low-fat cream cheese (2 Tbsp.)
Banana (1)
Orange juice (1/2 cup)
> **Calories 385**
> **Fat 2g**

Mini-bagels (2)
Fat-free cream cheese (2 Tbsp.)
Strawberry jam (2 tsp.)
Grapefruit juice (1/2 cup)
> **Calories 305**
> **Fat 1g**

Smoothie, made with:
- —orange/pineapple juice (1/2 cup)
- —banana, peach, or mango (1/2)
- —strawberry yogurt (1 carton)
- —ice cubes (5)

Graham crackers (2 whole)

Calories 300
Fat 4g

Chapter Four

Snacking for Fitness and Athletic Performance

BETWEEN JOBS, SCHOOL, AND WORKOUTS, many active people—especially those who pursue aggressive athletic goals—have every minute of their days filled. Early morning, lunch time, and evening workouts often crowd out regular meals. Breakfast becomes a commuting affair, lunch is replaced with quick snacks throughout the day, and dinner turns into late night munchies. Snacking plays an important role in fueling an active lifestyle and actually fits the schedules of many active people. Regardless of whether you are a competitive or recreational athlete, if you train or work out intensely on a regular basis, you have special nutrition needs that may be hard to meet with only three meals a day.

Why Athletes Need Snacks

As an athlete, your energy needs are higher than those who are not as active. Depending on your workout routine, you might need and extra 100 to 1,000 or more calories a day to supply the energy needed for exercise. For example, a woman who jogs three miles three times a week would need an extra 125 calories a day in addition to the 1,800 calories she needs for daily living. On the other hand, a woman training for a triathlon who has two endurance workouts a day, each lasting 45 minutes to an hour, might need 1,500 extra calories—close to double her maintenance calorie needs. Teenage athletes, who have increased energy needs due to growth as well as exercise, might require as much as 4,000 calories a day.

If you only need 500 extra calories or less, eating larger portions at meals can easily fill the gap. But if you need more than 3,000 calories a day, it can be hard to eat this much in three meals—eating over 1,000 calories in a single meal just before or immediately after a long workout can be uncomfortable. This is where snacking comes in. Well-chosen snacks can provide the fuel you need to sustain high levels of energy. Snacking is especially helpful if your schedule is so tight that you tend to skip a meal here and there. On the other hand, munching on high-fat and sweet treats such doughnuts, chips, and candy won't provide the best fuel for peak performance.

Fuel for Sports

Athletes, coaches, and exercise physiologists now know that exercise is not a license to overeat. It was once believed that if you exercised enough it didn't matter what or how much you ate. But experts now agree that the quality of the food you eat is as important as the quantity when fueling for performance.

Importance of Carbohydrates. Carbohydrates, fat, and protein provide energy in the form of calories. These three fuels each play different roles in the body, and all are used for exercise. Carbohydrates have one role: to provide energy for the muscles, brain, nerves, and other body tissues. Providing energy to fuel muscles is especially important for athletic performance. Protein is used for growth, maintenance, and repair of the body. As an athlete, you need protein to build muscles and heal both small and large wounds that result from strenuous exercise. Fat, both from food and from stored body fat, serves as an energy source, primarily for endurance-type exercise.

Interestingly, fats used during activity must "burn in a carbohydrate flame," meaning your body can only use fat as an energy source when carbohydrates are also being used for energy. For example, most people have enough fat stored in their bodies to run from New York City to Chicago, but only enough carbohydrates stored to run about 18 to 20 miles. The amount of available carbohydrates is the limiting factor in endurance performance. Therefore, carbohydrates are the most important fuel for athletes. A high-carbohydrate intake allows you to perform your best for a longer time. You can train harder and recover faster if you eat high-carbohydrate snacks and meals.

Fruits, vegetables, and grain products—foods from the base of the Food Guide Pyramid (page 5)—are your best snack food choices. They offer carbohydrates in addition to other valuable nutrients. Fruits and vegetables provide vitamins and minerals, such as vitamins A and C, potassium, and zinc. Vitamin C and zinc promote healing and protect against infection. Potassium, along with sodium and chloride, is lost in sweat. Enriched breads, cereals, crackers, and pasta supply iron, which is needed for carrying oxygen to your muscles. Iron deficiency can dramatically impair your performance.

Water. In addition to extra carbohydrates, you need more water. When you exercise for an hour or more, especially in hot and humid weather, you can lose a lot of fluids and become dehydrated. For example, a football player dressed in full gear could lose 3 quarts of water during an August training session. Runners, cyclists, rowers, baseball players, and virtually all competitive athletes face serious fluid losses during their training and competition.

Dehydration not only impairs performance, but it can be life threatening. Drinking fluids along with snacks is a good way to prevent dehydration. Water, juice, or sports drinks are the best choices. Caffeine-containing drinks, such as coffee, tea, and many soft drinks, promote fluid loss so they are not good fluid replacement drinks. Alcoholic beverages have the same dehydrating effect.

Snacks for Athletic Events and Workouts

Many athletes seek a miracle food or meal for the day of a big event, hoping to gain a competitive edge. In reality, nutritional conditioning goes hand-in-hand with physical conditioning. So, just as no special training technique done the day of an event will make up for months of inadequate training, no special food or meal can make up for months of poor eating. Meeting your nutrient needs throughout training is the only way to be nutritionally conditioned for a big event. Still, there are a few nutritional considerations that can fine-tune your performance during training and competition.

Before Exercise. Preferences of what to eat before exercise vary from person to person and sport to sport, so there is no single right choice. Most athletes learn through trial and error what works for them. When thinking through your choices, remember that snacks or meals eaten before exercise serve to:

- fill the carbohydrate stores in your muscles (this is especially important if you haven't eaten within the last four hours);
- prevent low blood sugar, which can cause light-headedness, blurry vision, poor concentration, and fatigue—all of which can limit your performance;
- settle your stomach by absorbing stomach juices and taking the edge off hunger;
- calm your jitters by knowing that your body is well-fueled.

When picking your snacks, consider how long it will be before you exercise. Food sitting in your stomach can slow you down and cause stomach cramps. Fat and protein take longer to digest, while carbohydrates are more quickly digested and absorbed, entering the bloodstream within 30 to 60 minutes. A high fiber content slows digestion and absorption. The size of the feeding will also affect how long it takes to digest—more calories means a longer digestion time.

When you're snacking shortly before exercise, steer away from high-fat foods and keep the portions small. Select high-carbohydrate foods such as English muffins, bagels, soda crackers, bread sticks, dry cereal, and rice cakes. They are easy to digest, settle your stomach, and keep your blood sugar level stable. A low-fat protein food can be added to your snack, especially if you haven't eaten for several hours. Try pairing low-fat dairy products with breads and cereals—bagels with fat-free cream cheese, cereal with nonfat milk, or a sandwich made from lean meat or poultry.

When snacking four or more hours before exercise, you have enough time to digest a mixture of protein, carbohydrates, and fat. For example, a snack of cheese and crackers with fresh fruit, cheese pizza, or tuna salad sandwich will curb your hunger longer. Depending on how much you eat, you may need a quick, carbohydrate snack a few hours later to top off your energy stores.

During Exercise. For exercise lasting less than 90 minutes, there is no need to eat during exercise. But, your performance in endurance events lasting longer than 90 minutes can be enhanced by drinking carbohydrate-containing fluids every 15 to 20 minutes during exercise. Solid foods take longer to be absorbed than fluids and can cause an upset stomach when consumed during exercise. Soft drinks are too concentrated and can draw water out of the body; plus the carbonation can cause stomach bloating and cramps. Sports drinks, on the other hand, are specially formulated for rapid absorption during exercise. Many athletes find them to be a convenient source of fluids and carbohydrates during exercise.

Solid food may be needed by athletes involved in sports that involve intermittent competitions over several hours. Snacking in between events may be the only way to keep fueled. For example, a person playing in a weekend handball or racquetball tournament may play several matches a day with only a few hours in between each. High-carbohydrate, low-fat snacks will boost energy stores without leaving a load in the stomach. Many other sports—soccer, hockey, swimming, track, gymnastics—also involve intense schedules during tournaments and meets. Well-timed snacks can prevent the stale feeling that sets in after several successive bouts of competition.

After Exercise. After a hard workout, your top priority should be to replace the fluids and electrolytes (sodium, potassium, and chloride) that you lost in sweat. To determine how much fluid you lost, weigh yourself before and after you exercise. For every pound of weight lost, you should drink at least one pint (two cups) of fluid. Water, fruit and vegetable juices, watery foods like watermelon or soup, sports drinks, or non-caffeinated soft drinks will all help to replace your water loss. Fruit or vegetable juices, sports drinks, and watery foods provide water, carbohydrates, and electrolytes. Soft drinks offer carbohydrates but no electrolytes, vitamins, or minerals.

A 20- to 30-minute workout won't deplete the carbohydrate stored in your muscles, but if you do two or more workouts a day or exercise for more than 90 minutes, you need to replace the stored carbohydrate that was used for exercise. Athletes at training camps who practice morning and afternoon, swimmers who compete in multiple events per day, triathletes who train twice a day, and aerobics instructors who teach several classes a day need to refuel before they exercise again. Your carbohydrate stores will recover faster if you eat within 1 to 4 hours after your workout.

Aim to consume half a gram of carbohydrates per pound of body weight (for example, 180 pounds x 0.5 grams = 90 grams) within 2 hours, and repeat this amount two hours later. It won't take much food to meet your needs; the following snacks provide about 45 to 50 grams of carbohydrate:

➤ a bagel and half cup of orange juice,

➤ a cup of cereal and half cup of nonfat milk,

➤ a carton of fruit yogurt,

➤ a whole graham cracker and half cup of pudding.

The Nutrition Facts label on food products can help you identify the carbohydrate content of foods. For more guidance on reading nutrition labels, refer to "A Lesson in Label Reading," page 8).

Smart Snacks for Athletes and Active People

Active people need convenient access to portable snacks they can eat quickly while pursuing other activities. A little advance planning can make it easier to keep healthy snacks on hand for when you need them. Identify high-carbohydrate, low-fat foods that you can pack or stash (refer to Appendix A for some ideas).

When eating less than two hours before a workout, select a single, high-carbohydrate food from the grain, fruit, or vegetable lists in Appendix A or a mini-meal that supplies 150 calories or less. Snacks eaten 3 to 4 hours before a workout can be larger (300 to 600 calories). Review the mini-meals in "Mini-Meals for Athletes" at the end of this chapter to get ideas for snacks that fit this range. After a long workout (90+ minutes), focus on replacing your fluids and carbohydrates with fruits, vegetables, grains, and beverages that supply at least 50 grams of carbohydrate per serving. During exercise, your appetite is suppressed and it may take a couple of hours after a long, strenuous workout for it to return to normal. Once you feel ready to eat again, try eating a combination of foods, such as the mini-meals beginning on page 45.

Promoting an Active Snacking Lifestyle

People on the go sometimes find that it is easier to snack than to eat regular, sit-down meals. This grazing approach to eating may work well for athletes who spend a lot of time training, but when eating on the run means unbalanced and inadequate nutrient intake, it can take a toll on your health and performance.

Case in point: Bill is a 40-year-old corporate executive with a wife and two children. He commutes to work 45 minutes each way, and is training for a marathon. During the week, Bill rises at 5:00 a.m., runs five or six miles, gets ready for work, and catches a commuter train at 6:45 a.m. There is no time to sit down for breakfast. Sometimes he grabs a muffin or doughnut and coffee on the way to the office. He either skips lunch or munches on microwave popcorn at his desk—unless he has a business luncheon. When Bill gets home at 7:00 p.m., he is fatigued and famished. After a substantial dinner, he snacks on chips, cookies, and ice cream to soothe the tension in his stomach. On Saturdays, he runs at least 10 miles, gradually building his mileage as he approaches the marathon. Four months into his training, Bill starts to feel stale and then comes down with a cold he can't shake. Clearly, Bill's demanding schedule and haphazard eating patterns have caught up with him.

Snacking on several healthy mini-meals throughout the day will fit Bill's schedule and improve his nutrient intake. All it takes is a little advanced planning. A bagel, yogurt, and orange tossed into his briefcase can be eaten on the train. This will provide carbohydrates, protein, calcium, and vitamin C, in contrast to the doughnut and coffee which only provided carbohydrates and a lot of fat. Emergency munchies could be stored in his desk drawer for nibbling throughout the day—dry cereal, bread sticks, rice cakes, low-fat crackers, pretzels, and dried fruit. Bill can grab yogurt or nonfat milk from a vending machine or run to the employee cafeteria for a sandwich or slice of pizza. With fresh fruit and vegetables from home, Bill can round off these snacks. These munchies will provide more nourishment than the microwave popcorn he's been choosing. At night, air- or stove-popped popcorn and frozen yogurt will make Bill's evening snack a lower fat indulgence. Also, by eating more during the day, he won't feel as compelled to snack at night.

Mini-Meals for Athletes

Pizza bagel (2 whole wheat bagel halves spread with 3 Tbsp.
  tomato paste or pizza sauce, sliced mushrooms (2 Tbsp.), sprinkled with 4 Tbsp. grated mozzarella cheese)
Baby carrots (3)
Apple juice (3/4 cup)
> **Calories 350**
> **Fat 7g**
> **Carbohydrate 60g**

Reduced fat chocolate sandwich cookies (2)

Nonfat milk (1 cup)

Apple (1 medium)

Calories 275
Fat 3g
Carbohydrate 54g

Fat-free whole wheat snack crackers (1 oz.)

Herbed cottage cheese dip, made from low-fat (1%) cottage cheese
(1/4 cup)

Carrot (1/2 whole) and celery sticks (1/2 stalk)

Mineral water

Calories 150
Fat 0.5g
Carbohydrate 24g

Trail mix (dry cereal, raisins, pretzels) (1 cup)

Low-fat fruit yogurt (1 cup)

Apple-raspberry juice (1 1/2 cups)

Calories 525
Fat 4g
Carbohydrate 113g

Baked potato, cooked in microwave for 10 minutes. Add your
choice of toppings and cook 2 to 3 minutes more:
—low-fat (1%) cottage cheese (1/4 cup)
—fat-free sour cream or yogurt (1/4 cup)

Raw cauliflower (1/2 cup) and baby carrots (3)

Ice water

Calories 200
Fat 1g
Carbohydrate 37g
Nutrient analysis based on cottage cheese

Graham crackers (2 whole)

Banana (1)

Fruit yogurt (1 cup)

Apple-cherry juice (1 cup)

Calories 590
Fat 6g
Carbohydrate 124g

Raisin bagel (1) with fat-free cream cheese (2 Tbsp.)

Apple (1)

Nonfat milk (1 cup)

Calories 435
Fat 2g
Carbohydrate 85g

Mini-bagels (2)

Fat-free cream cheese (2 Tbsp.)

Strawberry jam (2 tsp.)

Grapefruit juice (1/2 cup)

Calories 305
Fat 1g
Carbohydrate 60g

Smoothie, made with:

—orange/pineapple juice (1/2 cup)

—banana, peach, or mango (1/2)

—strawberry yogurt, low-fat (1 carton)

—ice cubes (5)

Graham crackers (2 whole)

Calories 300
Fat 4g
Carbohydrate 60g

Banana split made with

—banana (1)

—fat-free frozen strawberry yogurt (1 cup)

—strawberry topping (1 Tbsp.)

—nondairy whipped topping (1 Tbsp.)

Calories 365
Fat 2g
Carbohydrate 80g

Chapter Five

Snacking for the Weight Conscious

IF YOU'VE EVER TRIED to lose weight by skipping meals, you probably found that going for a long stretch without eating only made you ravenously hungry and more likely to overeat at your next meal. In fact, eating binges are common following a period of starvation or severe calorie restriction. One way to prevent this subsequent urge to overeat is to eat smaller amounts of food more frequently so you don't allow yourself to become too hungry. And careful food choices can keep your calorie intake in check while providing essential nutrients.

Lose Weight Not Nutrients

There is nothing magical or easy about losing weight. The bottom line is that you need to burn more calories than you consume. Exercise in addition to reducing food calories helps to tip the calorie equation in favor of weight loss.

Reducing Calories. Even though you eat fewer calories, your body still needs all the essential nutrients. This means that most of your calories should count nutritionally, leaving less room for the high-calorie, low-nutrient foods found at the top of the Food Guide Pyramid (page 5)—fats, sweets, and oils. Think of these foods as "empty calorie" or "luxury" foods. It's like making ends meet with a 25 percent pay cut—after you pay for all the essentials, there isn't much left for luxury purchases. Consider fat and sugar as luxuries that you'll need to budget when you're trying to lose weight. Target the recommended number of servings from each food group to meet your nutrient needs, but seek the lower fat and lower sugar choices in each group.

Don't be misled into thinking that low-fat also means low-calorie. Low-fat food products may have only a minimal calorie reduction. Many people equate fat with calories, so they automatically think low-fat is lower in calories and they eat larger portions. (See Chapter 1, page 11 for more on this snacking myth.)

Another common snacking problem stems from a tendency to underestimate portion sizes. Learning to estimate and control portions are important skills to master in weight management. The following tips can help you manage your portion sizes.

Use a smaller plate or bowl. This forces you to take smaller portions, yet you still feel like you're eating a full plate.

Don't "waist" food. You don't have to eat the whole order of French fries, bag of microwave popcorn, or granola bar just because that's the amount you were served. Indulge in a taste, save it for later or share it with a friend. It's still wasteful to eat food that you don't need, and the "waste" will end up on your waist.

Divide and share. If you can't bring yourself to throw food away, divide large portions and wrap up half. You can share it with someone else or save it for a later snack.

Store single portions. Make handy, pre-portioned snacks by storing food in single-serve containers. For example, when opening a box of snack crackers, look at the number of Servings Per Container, grab this number of zipper-sealing storage bags, and fill each with a serving of crackers. Take one bag and stuff the rest back into the cracker box; next time you want a snack all you have to do is grab a serving.

Quit the clean plate club. Stop eating when you're full, rather than when your plate is empty.

••
Snacking Pitfall: Large, Jumbo, and Super Size Servings

Portion sizes served in restaurants have become so large that it's easy to lose perspective on what is a reasonable serving size. If you eat what is served to you, you're probably eating several servings, thinking that it is only one. For example, a plate of pasta served in a restaurant usually equals about two cups which is four standard servings, not one. A 3-ounce serving of meat is about as large as a deck of cards, a bar of soap, or a cassette tape, but many portions of meat are two to three times that size. A scoop of butter, the size of ping pong ball, on top of pancakes is six times the standard 1 teaspoon serving size. About 12 to 16 potato chips make a serving, not half of a one-pound bag.

This is not to say that you should never eat more than a "standard" serving. When you're served a portion that is larger than standard, count the total number of servings and apply it to the recommended number of servings from the Food Guide Pyramid. Balancing these larger portions with your other food choices over the course of a day or several days helps to curb overall calorie intake. In fact, controlling your portion sizes is one of the most effective ways to slash calories. Scan the Nutrition Facts labels on food products for the serving size information (see page 9). Measure foods and practice visualizing the size of these servings. After a while, you will get a feel for reasonable amounts and be better able to judge what's served to you.

More Carbohydrates and Fiber. Weight loss does not mean less of everything. Eating more of some foods—those containing carbohydrates, fiber, and water—can actually help you lose weight. By helping to control your hunger, these foods help you resist the urge to splurge and eat too much. Carbohydrates are digested and gradually released into your bloodstream, providing a steady supply of energy, which helps to keep hunger at bay. Fiber further slows digestion and promotes a slow release of energy from food. Fiber, along with water, also fills your stomach, providing a satisfied feeling. Whole grain foods, fruits, and vegetables provide both carbohydrates and fiber. Many of these foods require crunching and chewing, which is a craving for many people who struggle with their weight (See Appendix C).

Water Flushes Toxins. More water is needed during weight loss to flush out toxins that are released when your body breaks down fat for energy. But some people mix up their thirst and hunger sensations and eat when they're actually thirsty. Emptiness in the stomach, headache, tiredness, and weakness are all signs of dehydration that could be mistaken for hunger. Learning to distinguish the difference between hunger and thirst is an important stepping stone in the path to lifelong weight control. Drinking more fluids and eating foods with a high water content can prevent dehydration along with the unpleasant sensations that can lead to unnecessary eating.

Fruits and vegetables, soups, and dairy products have a high water content. Because diet soft drinks, herbal teas, sparkling water, bottled mineral water, and tap water have no calories, they are also good fluid choices. Be aware, however, that the caffeine in coffee, tea, and many soft drinks stimulates hunger and causes your body to lose fluids, so they are not the best fluid choices. Fruit and vegetable juices are higher in calories, but they also provide vitamins and minerals. Alcoholic beverages have an effect similar to caffeine, plus they are high in calories. (Alcohol supplies 7 calories per gram, in contrast to the 4 calories per gram in carbohydrates and protein.)

Modifying Your Snacking Habits

Snacking was once forbidden fruit for dieters, but some snacking can actually aid weight loss by preventing hunger attacks. To use snacking to your advantage, first assess whether your snacking routines are conducive to weight loss. (Complete the Snacking Habits profile in Chapter 1, page 2.) Uncontrollable eating binges, mindless munching, and snacking on large amounts of empty-calorie foods are habits you need to modify if you are serious about losing weight and keeping it off.

Think about how snacking fits into your daily routine. The most popular time for snacking is during the evening when watching TV and winding down from the day. But morning and afternoon snack breaks also are common. Snacking can fit into any part of your day—as long as you tailor your food choices to fit the situation. Build your snacking strategies around when you like to snack. Then compare your average daily food choices to the Food Guide Pyramid (page 5) and select snacks to fill in where you may not typically meet the recommended number of servings. Stay on the lookout for the following snacking challenges and modify these routines.

Morning Blues. If you skip breakfast in exchange for a mid-morning snack, make your snack a hearty one. When you've gone more than 4 hours without eating, your body needs energy. Build your morning snack around a grain product, preferably whole grain. English muffins, bagels, bread, toast, cereal, or muffins are quick fixes in the morning. Adding a low-fat milk product, which will supply protein and calcium, is easy because of the variety of portable, single-serve dairy products available such as yogurt, nonfat milk, or pudding. Round off your snack with fruit to boost your carbohydrate, fiber, vitamin A, and vitamin C intake. For example, a whole wheat bagel, carton of low-fat fruit yogurt, and small banana will supply 500 calories and 4 grams of fat. Or try a cup of bran cereal with raisins and half cup of nonfat milk for 215 calories and 1 gram of fat.

If your mid-morning snack is in addition to breakfast, keep it light. Aim for a snack that is less than 100 calories, such as orange slices or rice cakes. Watch out for mindless munching routines—this is where the calories add up. Make your snack a deliberate choice that fits into your overall eating routine. It may be helpful to pre-portion your food and take a 3- to 5-minute break to eat it.

Mid-Afternoon Meltdown. It's 3:00 p.m., you're feeling drowsy, so you reach for a candy bar. No, wait! Dried fruit, crackers, pretzels, or celery or carrot sticks will supply more energy-boosting nutrients while satisfying your urge to chew. (Try the handy new snack packs of veggies with dip and pretzels or breadsticks.) However, if you're famished from skipping lunch, make your snack more substantial. A candy bar contains about the same calories and fat as a tuna sandwich, but none of the protein or B vitamins. Go for the sandwich—and add some fresh fruits or vegetables.

Evening Zone. Do you frequently find yourself winding down from a long day in front of the tube with a bag of chips close at hand? Stop! Have you eaten dinner yet? If not, think about what you're going to have and select a snack that nutritionally enhances the meal. For example, lead into a rich meal such as lasagna or beef stroganoff with fresh-cut vegetables. On the other hand, if you've already had dinner, those chips may be "waist-ful." If you're eating from boredom or stress, find something else to do with your hands. Eating the bulk of calories in one meal is associated with changes in metabolism that promote weight gain. This suggests that the pattern of calorie loading in the evening may not be conducive to weight management.

Snacking for the Weight Conscious

Smart Snacks for Weight Control

After looking at your snacking habits and identifying problem areas, think through ways to combat these problems. For example, substitute low-calorie crunchies for empty calorie foods during mindless munching episodes; the calorie impact of overdoing it is much less if you're eating carrots instead of potato chips. Prevent uncontrolled eating binges that stem from severe deprivation by eating small snacks throughout the day. And try to make snacking a planned activity, rather than an unconscious habit.

Winning snacks during weight loss are low in calories and rich in nutrients. Foods that are high in carbohydrates and fiber—grain products, fruits, and vegetables—help to curb hunger and binge eating. Satisfy your sensory cravings with lower fat and lower calorie snacks (Appendix C). Be aware that the hidden fat in many popular snack foods, such as crackers, cookies, chips, and muffins, make these foods high in calories, so keep the portions small. Take it easy on the high-fat partners that go with many high-carbohydrate foods, such as cream cheese on bagels and butter on popcorn. Or, try lowfat or fat-free cream cheese on a bagel or butter spray on popcorn.

Remember to drink fluids with your snacks. Reach for the low- or no-calorie drinks. Fill up on water, flavored water, diet drinks, or herbal teas. Fruit and vegetable juices are nutritious choices but the calories can add up quickly if juices are your primary fluid source.

When snacking replaces meals, turn your snacks into mini-meals by combining foods from different food groups. Think about how the snack fits with other foods you're eating that day and round off your mini-meals by filling in the missing gaps. For example, if you find that it is hard for you to eat at least five servings of fruits and vegetables a day, think about how you can pair fruits and vegetables with other snack foods.

Mini-Meals for the Weight Conscious

Fig bars, fat-free (2)
Nonfat milk (1 cup)
    Calories 220
    Fat 0.5g

Baked tortilla chips, low-fat (20 chips)
Salsa (1/4 cup)
Green and red peppers (1/2 cup)
    Calories 175
    Fat 5g

Fruit sundae made with:
   —fat-free frozen yogurt (1/2 cup)
   —frozen raspberries (1/4 cup)
   —low-calorie whipped topping (1 Tbsp.)
    Calories 155
    Fat 0.5g

Hard pretzels, Dutch twist (2 large)
Spicy mustard (1 Tbsp.)
Sparkling mineral water
    Calories 140
    Fat 2.5g

Angel food cake (1 piece/53g)
Fresh strawberries (1/2 cup)
Low-calorie whipped topping (1 Tbsp.)
Decaffeinated coffee or tea, black
    Calories 165
    Fat 1g

Tortilla wrap (roll lean deli-sliced turkey (1 oz.), shredded lettuce
    (2 Tbsp.), diced tomatoes (2 Tbsp.), and fat-free mayonnaise
    (2 tsp.) in a flour tortilla)
Diet soft drink
    Calories 155
    Fat 3g

Raisin bagel (1) with fat-free cream cheese (2 Tbsp.)
Orange (1 medium)
    Calories 285
    Fat 1.5g

Whole wheat English muffin (1) with apple butter (2 tsp.)
Hot herbal tea
    Calories 150
    Fat 1g

Chapter Six
Snacking
at Work

DOUGHNUTS BY THE DOZENS, monthly birthday cakes, desktop candy jars, happy hour buffets, vending machine treats, and fundraiser goodies make many worksites a snacking obstacle course. Since work consumes a lot of your time, it is important to explore ways to make your worksite snacking habits healthy. Although you can't change the culture of the worksite or force your coworkers to change the way they eat, you can control your food choices and eating habits by:
> ➤ bringing healthy snacks to work,
> ➤ preventing yourself from becoming too hungry,
> ➤ selecting healthy foods when planning meetings and social events.

Worksite Snacking Habits
Cola to wake up...doughnuts to settle in to the day...pretzels to proofread...cookies to collate...candy to relieve boredom. Do you associate the tasks of your workday with nibbles and munchies that have become part of your daily routine? For some people, snacking while working is second nature. For others, snacks are confined to scheduled breaks. Others grab snacks at work in a fit of hunger because they have skipped breakfast or lunch. Let's explore some common worksite snacking habits and ways to improve them.

Desktop Dining. From the goody jar on top of the desk to candy stashes in the drawers to brown bag lunches, many desks serve as much food as kitchen tables. If eating at your desk is a purposeful activity—eating a meal or planned snack—and it doesn't interfere with your work responsibilities, then desktop dining can be an efficient way to meet your calorie and nutrient needs. On the other hand, if you nibble mindlessly and lose sight of what you've eaten or how much, it's time to curb the habit. Trade the candy jar for a fruit bowl and stash pretzels or rice cakes in your drawers so your mindless munching makes a nutritional contribution without the calorie damage.

Savory Breaks. If you work a structured schedule you probably look forward to your breaks. Socializing with co-workers, nibbling on a tasty treat, and a brief escape from the monotony of the job make breaks an appealing part of the day. Although eating during a break may be second nature, take a moment to think about whether you really need food at this time of day and how it fits into your overall eating pattern. For example, a mid-morning break is a good time to make up for a skipped breakfast. But rather than doughnuts and coffee, select a low-fat bread or cereal and add a fruit and dairy product. If you've already eaten breakfast, keep the mid-morning snack light with rice cakes, fruit, or the like. Better yet, pursue nonfood activities during your breaks, such as walking, shopping, reading, or running an errand.

Power Meetings. Pastries and coffee in the morning and cookies and soft drinks in the afternoon. These are the typical offerings served at many corporate meetings to break the ice and promote fellowship. These unexpected snacks may replace or supplement your regular meals and snacks, resulting in nutritional imbalances or extra calories and fat. At your worksite, talk to the person in charge of ordering food and suggest bagels and fruit instead of (or in addition to) doughnuts, high-fat muffins, and cookies. Arrange for diet soft drinks, bottled mineral water, and sparkling water to be served with regular soft drinks. When you are a guest, either graciously decline an offer of food or take half a doughnut or cookie.

Coffee Club. Many worksites have a pot of coffee brewing all day long. It's easy to slip into the habit of starting the day at the coffee station, visiting with coworkers and taking a mug to your desk as you settle into work. This morning mug can easily turn into an all-day habit of sipping a cup an hour, or 8 to 10 cups a day. This amount of caffeine can make you jittery, distracted, and nervous. Eventually you'll find yourself hooked on caffeine and unable to function without a daily dose. Caffeine also stimulates the release of stomach juices, which triggers hunger feelings. You might notice this sensation as a "churning or gurgling in your stomach." Because it feels similar to hunger sensations, for some people it may lead to needless snacking. Plus, if you add sugar and creamer to every cup of coffee, you could be consuming an extra 400 to 500 calories. Try to limit your caffeinated coffee to two cups a day and use nonfat creamer, nonfat milk, and sugar substitutes.

Making Your Food Choices Work

Sorting through the various food choices at work takes a little thought and skill. Although many typical food venues—vending machines, cafeterias, and food carts—serve many high-calorie, high-fat, or nutritionally empty foods, you can be selective about what you choose.

Vending Machines. The vending machine is most tempting when you're hungry, have no other food handy, and have no time to wander out to the deli or cafeteria. Although vending foods come in small sizes, don't be misled. The small bags of chips, tiny packs of cookies, and miniature cheese and cracker packs are often big on calories and fat. The convenience of vending machines cannot be ignored; there are times when a vending machine snack can tide you over or supplement your desk drawer stash. Seek the foods that are lower in calories and fat. For example, pretzels are almost always available in vending machines.

Vending Machine Snacks

	Fat (grams)	Calories
Candy bars (1)	13	280
Cheese curls (1 oz.)	24	320
Chewing gum (1 stick)	0	15
Corn chips (1 oz.)	9	155
Crackers, cheese & peanut butter (4)	7	135
Fresh fruit (1 medium)	0	60
Apple juice (6 fl. oz. can)	0	80
Hard candies (1 oz.)	0	105
Licorice (1 oz.)	0.5	105
Low-fat fruit yogurt (8 oz. carton)	3	250

	Fat (grams)	Calories
Microwave popcorn (1/2 bag)	12	220
Potato chips (1 oz.)	10	150
Pretzels (1 oz.)	1	110
Raisins (1 oz.)	0	85
Sandwich cookies (4)	8	190
Soft drinks, diet (12 fl. oz. can)	0	0
Soft drinks, regular (12 fl. oz. can)	0	150

Delis and Cafeterias. Many worksites are offering healthier fare in their employee cafeterias, posting nutrition information, or featuring a "wellness menu." These programs make it easier than it once was to select healthier foods at work. When you visit the cafeteria for breakfast or lunch, grab an extra piece of fruit for your morning or afternoon break. Bagels, miniature boxes of cereal, and single-serve containers of nonfat milk and fruit juice can be carried to your desk on days you missed breakfast. Low-fat sandwiches can be made to order from the deli counter for a late lunch or mid-afternoon snack. Go easy on fried foods, high-fat dressings and sauces, cookies and ice cream, and fatty deli meats to keep your snacks low in fat and calories.

Best Picks for Delis and Carry-Outs

Breads and cereals

Select More Often

Bagel	Pita bread
Bran cereal	Pumpernickel bread
Dry cereal, unsweetened	Rye bread
English muffin	Whole wheat bread
Kaiser roll	

Select Less Often

Croissant	Doughnuts
Granola	Muffins (most are high-fat)
Danish roll	Pastries

Sandwich fillings

Select More Often

Chicken breast	Low-fat hot dogs
Lean ham	Turkey breast
Lean roast beef	Turkey dogs

Bacon	Hot dog
Bologna	Meatballs
Bratwurst	Pastrami
Braunschweiger	Pepperoni
Cheese	Salami
Chicken salad	Sausage
Deviled ham	Tuna salad

Sandwich toppings and sauces

Select More Often

Catsup	Low-fat dressing
Green pepper	Mustard
Hot peppers	Sauerkraut
Lemon juice	Tomato
Lettuce	Vinegar

Select Less Often

Guacamole	Oil
Dressing, regular	Olives
Mayonnaise	

Food Carts. A combination concession stand and vending machine, these mobile units appear outside office buildings and busy pedestrian walkways at convenient times of the day. Because most of the food is already prepared and wrapped, you can't make any special requests to skip the mayonnaise or hold the bacon. The hot dogs are not likely to be the low-fat variety, and the sandwiches usually are loaded with mayonnaise. But you may be able to score some smart snacks at these roving counters, such as low-fat yogurt, fresh fruit, plain bagels, fruit juice, and nonfat milk.

Creating Healthy Food Stashes

The best way to guarantee that you have healthy foods available at work is to bring food with you. Having your own snacks will make it easier to resist the vending machine treats, birthday cake, and plates of doughnuts around the office. Stashing food at work also will save you money since it's much cheaper to purchase foods at a supermarket than a convenience store, cafeteria, or vending machine. Add single-serve containers of cereal, pudding, canned fruit, crackers, juice boxes, and snack kits to your weekly grocery list. Many of these foods are available in variety- or multi-packs. Take inventory of your worksite stashes once a week, noting what you want to restock and disposing of old and spoiled food. Don't forget to store utensils that you'll need to prepare and eat the food you've stashed.

Worksite Food Stashes

Cold Storage

Baby carrots	Mineral or sparkling water
Convenience snack packs	Sandwiches
Fresh cut mixed vegetables	Nonfat milk
Fresh fruit	String cheese
Juice boxes	Yogurt, low-fat or nonfat

Dry Storage

Applesauce (single-serve)	Low-fat cookies (fig bars, ginger
Baked chips	snaps, vanilla wafers)
Canned or dried fruit	Low-fat microwave popcorn
Canned or dehydrated soup	Peanut butter
Dry cereal	Pretzels
Instant oatmeal packets	Pudding (single-serve)
Low-fat crackers (graham crackers,	Rice cakes
soda, whole grain)	Tuna (single-serve can)

Utensils

Bowl (microwaveable)	Sharp knife
Can opener	Spoon, fork, butter knife
Plate (use as cover for bowl)	Storage bags
Pre-moistened wipes	

Cold Storage. Many worksites have a refrigerator for perishable items. Communal refrigerators quickly can become disorganized and laden with spoiled food. Everyone needs to do their part to keep track of their food and discard old food before it spoils. Label your foods with your name and date to help you keep tabs on what you've got in storage.

If you don't have access to a refrigerator, you can pack foods in an insulated lunch bag with a frozen cold pack. For those who work out of their vehicles, cold food can be stored in a portable container.

Dry Storage. Non-perishable foods can be stashed in a desk drawer, locker, or glove compartment. Designate a drawer of your desk or file cabinet or use your locker for storing dry goods. Crackers, soups, pretzels, rice cakes, and pudding make great snacks or building blocks for mini-meals. Be sure to keep food well wrapped and clean up crumbs on a regular basis so you don't attract bugs and other pests.

Lunch Box Munchies. If you pack a lunch, toss in a few extra items for snacking. Fresh fruit, rice cakes, pretzels, low-fat snack crackers, dried fruit, dry cereal, or low-fat yogurt are easy additions to a lunch box. If you don't feel like eating them during your workday, add them to your stash.

Chapter Seven

Snacking at Home

NOT LONG AGO, families gathered together for three meals a day. These days, two-career families, single-parent families, children's extracurricular activities, and single-person homes have made this lifestyle impractical or impossible. Eating routines around the home might involve a breakfast of cereal with milk eaten alone by each family member and maybe a family dinner, with the remainder of eating consisting of random snacking by whomever is hungry. Because of the varied and hectic schedules of today's households, healthy snacking can serve as a practical alternative to the traditional, three-square-meals-a-day routine.

Daytime Nibbles

Parents who stay home with young children, retirees, telecommuters, home-based entrepreneurs, night-shift workers, and other people who spend their days at home have ready access to the cupboard throughout the day. Tasty desserts left from the night before look tempting on a pass through the kitchen. Cookie jars and candy bowls offer treats for the taking. Ice cream is only a scoop away. Potato chips..."I'll just have one."

Snacking relieves boredom for some people. Others have gotten into the habit of snacking while doing other activities, such as watching TV or surfing the net. Taking snack breaks can be a way to put off unpleasant tasks, like vacuuming, dusting, or laundry. Those who care for small children can get drawn into snacking every time they serve food to the kids, which can be every two to three hours.

If your daytime snacking habits help to nutritionally balance your diet, hold on to them. (To assess your diet, compare your intake to the recommended servings from the Food Guide Pyramid, Chapter 1, page 5.) On the other hand, if your snacking routines are a source of excess calories and fat, you might benefit from some changes. Consider the following strategies:

Curb Mindless Munching. Zero in on situations where snacking has become an unconscious habit. Pay closer attention to how much you eat during these times and identify how you can make modifications. For example, substitute pretzels or celery for chips. Put a single serving of snacks into a bowl, rather than eating out of the bag.

Take Stock. Go through your cupboards, refrigerator, and freezer to assess the type of snacks you have on hand. Replace the high-calorie, low-nutrient foods with healthier choices. Compare your diet to the Food Guide Pyramid and identify if you need to boost your intake of any food groups. Stock up on these foods, so the next time you're scavenging for a snack, you'll find choices that make a nutritional boost.

Evening Snack Attacks

Before, after, or in place of dinner, evening is the most common time to snack. For many, snacking is a way to unwind from a stressful day. Others have been too busy to eat much all day and may be ready to devour everything in sight. People who don't know how to cook, or don't like to, find that heavy snacking is easier than eating dinner.

If snacking is in addition to dinner, keep your food choices light. But if snacking replaces dinner, make your snack substantial and nutritionally complete. Keep the following strategies in mind as you plan your evening snacking.

Tackle the Hunger Attack. Before-dinner snacks should be low in calories and fat so they don't ruin your appetite. Even if you're ravenously hungry, you're better off filling up on dinner than snacks. Raw vegetables, bread sticks, fat-free crackers, or pretzels will tide you over without filling you up. Cheese and crackers or chips and dip are fine in small amounts but incur a higher calorie cost.

Pause and Digest. After dinner, wait a few hours for your meal to digest before snacking. When you keep eating on a full stomach, you lose touch with your body's signals of hunger and fullness, making it easier to overeat all the time. Pay attention to your body's natural hunger cycles. You need food about every three to four hours, so if you eat dinner at 6:00 p.m., you may be ready for a snack at 9:00 or 10:00. Use your late-night snack as an opportunity to polish off your day. For example, if you've been light on milk products, frozen yogurt or pudding would be a good way to end the day.

Unwind Without Snacks. Snacking to relax and unwind can easily become a mindless munching game in which you eat more than you realize. Try to find other activities to relieve your stress, such as brisk walking, taking a hot bath, or listening to peaceful music. Eating meals and snacks throughout the day is a first-line defense against the late-night munchies. Going too long without food triggers deep-rooted survival instincts which drive you to overeat the next time you eat. Therefore if you haven't eaten all day (or eaten very little), you are more likely to overeat in the evening. If you find that you can't break this snacking habit, choose very low-calorie foods for your munchies. Celery sticks and rice cakes offer a lot of crunch for a few calories. Air- or stove-popped popcorn served without butter is another reasonable choice. Refer to Appendix C for more ideas to satisfy your sensory cravings without excess fat and calories.

Snack for Dinner. When snacking replaces dinner, build your snack into a mini-meal (see "Building Blocks of Healthy Snacking" in Chapter 1). Don't fall into the trap of eating a huge portion of one food and calling it dinner. For example, a whole bag of chips or box of cookies may provide 1,000 or more calories and make you feel full, but they won't supply other essential nutrients. Combine foods from different food groups, using the Food Guide Pyramid as a guide (page 5).

Serving Snacks to Guests

When the gang comes over for a Super Bowl party, you host your card club, or you throw a New Year's Eve bash, what kind of snacks do you serve? Choose snacks that have both crowd appeal and good nutrition. Crunchy foods are popular, so look for low-fat crunchies, such as baked tortilla chips, pretzels, low-fat seasoned crackers, and popcorn. Arrange the crunchy snacks with other foods that boost the nutritional profile. For example, serving tortillas with green, red, and yellow peppers and salsa adds fiber and vitamin C. By balancing these nutrition-packed choices with higher fat and calorie choices, you can provide your guests with a full range of options.

Light on the Hors D'oeuvres. Keep hors d'oeuvres light and simple. Make colorful displays with fresh fruits and vegetables—they whet but don't drench the appetite. Complement the fruit and vegetable platters with low-fat crackers. For an elegant affair, serve shrimp cocktail. At more casual functions, salsa and chips, pretzels, and popcorn make low-calorie nibbles.

Skinny on the Toppings and Spreads. Make spreads and dips with low-fat or fat-free yogurt, sour cream, cream cheese, and cottage cheese. These ingredients turn a snack of crackers and chips into a source of calcium and protein.

Heavy on the Vegetables and Grains. Think creatively about how to blend vegetables and grains into your snack food offerings. Serve pita triangles with hummus or other low-fat spreads. Stuff celery sticks and green pepper boats with a seasoned fat-free cream cheese spread. Fill a round loaf of sour dough bread with a healthy version of spinach dip made from low-fat mayonnaise and fat-free sour cream.

Lean on the Meat and Cheese. Cocktail meatballs, spicy sausage, cheese and cracker platters, and cheese balls rolled in nuts can amount to loads of calories and fat. Try using lean meats and low-fat cheeses. Cut full-fat meats and cheeses in thin slices or miniature-size pieces. Blend them with other foods, so the proportions are more like a condiment.

Generous on the Fruitful Treats. Serve desserts and treats that center around a fruit. Feature strawberries and low-fat yogurt with angel food cake. Skewer cubes of fresh fruit on tooth picks to make fruit kebabs and accompany them with a fruit purée made by blending frozen raspberries or strawberries.

Smart Snacks to Keep on Hand

The best way to control your snacking habits at home is to keep healthy snacks on hand. If you find that chips jump out of the cupboard faster than rice cakes, you might need to rearrange the shelves to make the healthier choice more accessible. You could also divide the package into single-serve portions which will help you control your portions. Better yet, when the chips and cookies are gone, don't buy replacements, or only allow yourself to buy these treats once in a while, such as once per month. You can make changes gradually, weaning yourself from high-fat and high-calorie treats, or do it in one clean sweep, clearing the cupboards and refrigerator of foods you can't resist overeating. Use whichever approach works best for you.

Review the food lists in Appendix A to identify smart snacks that might work for you. Put these on your grocery list and make a point of keeping them on hand.

Chapter Eight

Snacking on the Go

TODAY, MANY OF US eat on the run, munching while we drive, walk, work, and play. Single-serve portions, drive-through restaurants, take-out foods, and microwave meals make it easier than ever to grab a mouthful and go. This trend can be a problem if the foods are high in fat and calories, which is often the case. Let's look at some of the ways to eat healthfully on the go. Find one that fits your lifestyle.

Dashboard Dining

Sales representatives, service technicians, delivery staff, and truck drivers spend many hours behind the wheel. For some, erratic schedules make snacking in their vehicles the most convenient eating pattern. Others find that snacking relieves the boredom and monotony of driving. For families traveling with small children, snacking serves as a handy distraction and keeps food stops to a minimum. Convenience stores, fast food restaurants, diners, and coffee shops can get old when you're on the road a lot. The solution: stash healthy snacks in your vehicle. This will broaden your choices and save you time and money.

Vehicles can get very hot in the summer, so you need to be careful about storing foods that will melt, get messy, or taste bad when hot. Stick to dry foods such as crackers, rice cakes, and pretzels in hot weather or store foods like raisins or peanut butter in a cooler. Because glove compartments get extremely hot, don't stash food in them in hot weather—instead use a plastic storage container to keep foods organized and out of sight. Use a portable cooler to keep foods cold and prevent spoilage. Dry ice packs stay cold longer and are not as messy as ice cubes. Buy a couple of packs and rotate them from your freezer to your cooler.

When packing foods for the road, prepare them so they are ready to eat. For example, peel and slice an orange so that you're not wrestling with the peel while maneuvering through traffic. And combine dry foods with wet foods to prevent cotton mouth. Peanut butter is a classic example of a food that is hard to eat without something to wash it down—eat it with orange slices or a beverage. Good picks for dashboard dining:

➤ are single-serve,

➤ won't spill or make a mess,

➤ can be eaten with one hand,

➤ don't require utensils or preparation.

Packing for the Road

Cooler

Baby carrots	Mineral or sparkling water
Convenience snack packs	Sandwiches
Fresh cut vegetables	Nonfat milk
Fresh fruit	Yogurt, low-fat
Juice boxes	

Dry Storage

Canned or dried fruit	Peanut butter
Canned or dehydrated soup	Pretzels
Dry cereal	Pudding (single-serve)
Low-fat crackers	Rice cakes
Low-fat microwave popcorn	Trail mix

Commuting Crunch

Many people who live in large metropolitan areas often spend a couple hours a day commuting to work, either by train or car. The daily commute eats into time otherwise used for sleep, exercise, eating regular meals, relaxing, spending time with families, and recreation. Meals, especially breakfast, often take the brunt of the commuting time crunch. Using the commute for healthy snacking can make up for meals that are squeezed out.

Whether you drive or take the train, throw a few single-serve foods into your briefcase, purse, or knapsack to eat on your way to work. For example, a bagel and banana can be eaten with one hand and won't make crumbs or slop down the front of your clothes. When making your selections, go for:

- ➤ foods that won't spill or make a mess
- ➤ foods that can be eaten with your hands
- ➤ ready-to-eat foods
- ➤ combination of moist foods and dry foods

If you forget to pack food, swing into a drive-through restaurant for a glass of orange juice and English muffin before you board the train. Or make a quick stop at a food cart for a bagel, yogurt, and fruit on your walk to the office.

Commuting Cuisine

Mini-Breakfast Ideas

Bagel	Muffin, low-fat
Banana	Orange slices
Coffee/tea	Rice cakes
Fruit bar	Yogurt, low-fat
Juice box	

Snack Ideas

Apple	Granola bar
Banana	Mineral water
Diet soft drink	Pretzels
Dry cereal	Rice cakes
Grapes	Snack crackers, low-fat
Graham crackers	

Convenience Stop

Once considered a nutritional mine field, convenience stores have started to cater to health-conscious people on the go. Many stores now feature a healthy snack section, displaying low-fat and fat-free snack foods. Healthier versions of traditional snacks sit next to their high-fat and high-calorie cousins. Gourmet coffee, fruit-flavored iced tea, and sports drinks reflect the upscale tastes of today's consumer. On your way to the health food section, don't get sidetracked by the candy bars, chips, snack pies, doughnuts, and pastries.

Fast Food Feast

With the lines between a meal and a snack blurring in today's lifestyle, fast food restaurants offer snack, as well as meal, options. Open day and night with drive-up windows, they are a convenient stop for busy people. Though traditional fast foods mean fat and calories, there is a new wave of fast food choices which offer healthy alternatives.

When ordering fast foods, keep these strategies in mind:

Steer away from fried food. Chicken and fish may sound healthy, but once they are fried, the fat level soars.

Head for the salad bar. Be aware that many salad dressings and creamy salads, such as macaroni and potato, are high in fat.

Turn to potatoes with caution. A baked potato sounds innocent enough, but when you add the cheese, sour cream, bacon bits, or chili, the calories can easily triple and the fat level quickly rises.

Hold the cheese. Save the calories and fat for another meal or snack. Get your calcium from nonfat milk.

Think small or regular size. Double, triple, deluxe, super, extra, and jumbo spell fat and calories in capital letters.

Go easy on the sauces. Mayonnaise, special sauces, and tartar sauce are high in fat and calories. If the food is served with these toppings, scrape some off.

Best Snacks in Fast Food Restaurants

When Buying Breakfast, Order...

Bagel (with jam)
Canadian Bacon
English Muffin (with jam)
Fat-Free Muffin
Pancakes (with syrup, applesauce, or fruit)

When Buying Sandwiches, Order...

Fajita Sandwich
Grilled Chicken Sandwich
Plain Hamburger
Roast Chicken Sandwich
Roast Turkey Sandwich
Small Roast Beef Sandwich
Turkey Submarine

When Buying Potatoes & Other Side Dishes, Order...

Broth-Based Soups
Corn-on-the-Cob
Plain Baked Potato
Salads
Small Chili

When Buying Desserts, Order...

Low-Fat Milkshake	Non-Fat Frozen Yogurt
Low-Fat Yogurt Shake	Small Soft-Serve Cone

Jet Set Snacking

Some sales representatives, consultants, executives, and many professionals spend more time in airports and hotels than they do at home. Crossing time zones and crazy flight schedules can lead to skipped meals and heavy snacking at odd hours. And you can't rely on airlines for your meals—many have cut back their food service to snacks and beverages, except for transcontinental or overseas flights. On these longer flights, order special meals which are healthier—and sometimes tastier—than regular meals. Most airlines offer diabetic, low-cholesterol, low-sodium, heart-healthy, seafood, or vegetarian meals. Eating in flight will keep you from arriving at your hotel too hungry and attacking the mini-bar. Pack some light-weight snacks to supplement the airplane food (for example, rice cakes, pretzels, single-serve cereal boxes, raisin boxes, or dried fruit).

Snacks served in flight may be as simple as a beverage and bag of peanuts, or something more substantial such as a sandwich basket with chips, fruit, and cookies. Pass on the peanuts; take pretzels when you have the choice. Be picky with the snack basket—you don't have to eat everything. Think about how the snack fits with what else you're eating that day. If you've eaten breakfast and lunch, and you're planning to attend a dinner meeting, take the fruit and return the rest to the flight attendant. On the other hand, if you've missed meals earlier in the day and know you'll arrive too late for a decent meal, eat the whole snack. It will prevent you from becoming too hungry and overeating later.

Take advantage of the beverage service. Air travel saps water from your body, causing fatigue, light-headedness, and headaches. Replacing the fluids you lose will help you recover from jet lag and awaken the next day fresh and alert. Aim for one glass of water for every hour in flight. Beverages with alcohol and caffeine are dehydrating, so go easy on these beverages.

The airport waiting game can make even a patient person restless and bored. Many people seek tasty treats and comfort foods to relieve boredom and tension. If you are an occasional traveler, these

Snacking on the Go

splurges are no big deal, but if you travel frequently, it's not a wise habit to develop. Scope the airport for healthy choices. In larger airports, you can find a wide variety of foods and restaurants; however, the most convenient and common airport food venues are concession stands and cafeterias. Usually, they serve fresh fruit, bagels, and yogurt you can grab for your plane ride or eat during a layover. Better yet, fill your time with a good book or catch up on work, instead of snacking needlessly.

If you miss eating in flight and at the airport, and arrive at your hotel too late for restaurant dining, your choices are limited: room service, the hotel gift shop, or the mini-bar. That's why carrying travel snacks is a good preventive measure. Steer clear of the easy options, such as candy bars, chips, and nuts in the mini-bar or gift shop. Scan the room service menu for a salad or soup with a dinner roll. If the late-night menus only consists of burgers and other fried foods, ask if they will serve you a light, simple meal from another menu. For example, they may accommodate a request for dry cereal, nonfat milk, and fresh fruit even though it's not breakfast time.

Chapter Nine
Special Snacking Needs

SNACKING IS VERY IMPORTANT for certain people with special nutrition needs because of a health or disease condition. For example, a person with diabetes or hypoglycemia needs to eat frequently to help regulate blood sugar level. Snacking also is an effective way to boost calorie intake if you need to gain weight. Because most of the information in this book is geared to the needs of people who can benefit from snacks that are lower in calories and fat, this chapter addresses the special needs of people with diabetes, hypoglycemia, or a need to gain weight.

Diabetes
If you have diabetes, snacks are an important part of your meal plan. For people with Type 1 diabetes, snacks help to prevent large fluctuations in blood sugar levels. Between-meal and bedtime snacks are built into your meal plan to cover the peak times of insulin activity and physical activity. It is very important to eat these snacks on schedule to prevent a hypoglycemic reaction. Your meal plan is devised to match the size of the snack with the timing of the insulin activity—larger snacks are paired with the peak times of insulin activity. If you experience a hypoglycemic reaction, eat a snack with 15 grams of carbohydrate, wait 15 minutes (the "15/15 rule"), and retest your blood sugar.

Quick Carbohydrates:
Foods Containing Approximately 15 grams of Carbohydrate

Food	Serving Size
Ice cream	1/2 cup
Cooked cereal	1/2 cup
Sherbet	1/4 cup
Jello	1/3 cup
Broth-based soup, reconstituted	1 cup
Cream soup	1 cup
Carbonated soft drinks containing sugar	3/4 cup (6 fluid ounces)
Milkshake	1/4 cup
Milk	1/2 cup
Eggnog	1/2 cup
Tapioca pudding	1/3 cup
Custard	1/2 cup
Yogurt, plain	1 cup
Toast	1 slice
Soda crackers	6 crackers

For those with Type 2 diabetes who are not insulin-dependent, snacks provide a way to distribute calories evenly during the day to help the body's insulin work more effectively and to keep blood sugar levels more stable. Eating smaller meals with between-meal snacks also can help you control your appetite, making weight maintenance or loss easier. Many people who are able to lose weight find that their blood sugar control improves naturally.

Hypoglycemia
Many people incorrectly think they suffer from hypoglycemia, which is a condition of low blood sugar caused by hormone imbalances. Low blood sugar can happen to anyone who goes for an extended period without eating. Many vital organs, such as the brain and nervous system, depend on a steady supply of sugar to keep functioning. When blood sugar wanes, the result is a feeling of lightheadedness and low energy. For the average person, eating regular meals will prevent low blood sugar. However, about 5 percent of the population suffers from hypoglycemia caused by an overproduction of insulin or an underproduction of glucagon, hormones that regulate blood sugar. The symptoms include shakiness, sweating, rapid heartbeat, and trembling about two to four hours after eating. These

people need to take special dietary measures to control their blood sugar level.

Frequent snacks are important for managing hypoglycemia to prevent large drops in blood sugar levels. Each snack should include some protein, fat, and carbohydrates to create a slow, steady release of energy into the blood. The mini-meal approach to snacking will accomplish this goal (page 6). High fiber foods help to slow the absorption of sugar into the bloodstream. Alcoholic beverages and caffeine exaggerate the hypoglycemic effect, so they are best avoided.

Weight Gain

People suffering from cancer, AIDS, or anorexia may have a hard time gaining weight or preventing weight loss. A poor appetite, dry or sore mouth, and nausea may make it uncomfortable or impossible to eat larger meals. Therefore, adding several snacks a day is the most realistic approach to boosting calorie intake.

Adequate protein and calories (energy) are needed to prevent muscle tissue from being broken down as an energy source and to promote weight gain. Carbohydrates are a good source of energy, and they spare muscle protein from being used as an energy source. Because fat is a concentrated source of calories, snacks for people who need to gain weight can be higher in fat than what is recommended for an average adult. High-calorie, low-nutrient snacks, such as candy and chips, do not provide the nourishment your body needs to heal and fight infections. Select basic foods from the Food Guide Pyramid (page 5) and find creative ways to make them higher in calories. Refer to the next page for strategies to increase the calorie content of snacks.

Peanut butter, cottage cheese, and cheese are high-protein and high-fat foods that combine easily with fruits and grains. These food combinations create healthy snacks that are high in calories and packed with essential nutrients. Adding powdered milk to recipes is another effective way to increase the calories and protein. For example, blend a half cup of dry milk into a meatloaf or quick bread recipe. Combinations of fruit, yogurt or ice cream, and milk blended until smooth make high-calorie, nutritious drinks. Milk powder will further increase the calories and protein in these drinks.

Increasing the Calorie Content of Snacks

Breads, Cereals, Rice, and Pasta

➤ Select higher calorie breads, such as banana and cinnamon bread, muffins.

➤ Select regular snack crackers.

➤ Spread cream cheese and peanut butter on breads and crackers.

➤ Add nuts and raisins to cereal.

➤ Blend cottage cheese and apple butter to make a spread for crackers and bagels or stuffing for pita pockets.

➤ Make sandwiches with meat, cheese, egg salad, chicken salad, peanut butter. Add mayonnaise.

➤ Make toppings for popcorn from melted peanut butter, grated cheese, caramel.

➤ Combine various cheeses and snack crackers.

➤ Select or prepare a trail mix made with dry cereal, nuts, pretzels, and dried fruit.

➤ Roll up tortillas with melted cheese and refried beans.

Fruits

➤ Spread peanut butter on apple or pear slices.

➤ Mix applesauce with cottage cheese and raisins.

➤ Mash bananas with peanut butter to make a spread.

➤ Serve cottage cheese with cantaloupe, pineapple, or peaches.

➤ Mix dried fruit with nuts.

➤ Blend raisins, nuts, and candy-coated chocolates.

➤ Serve strawberries on top of angel food cake or short cake with a dollop of whipped cream or fruit yogurt.

Vegetables

➤ Top broccoli or cauliflower with grated cheese or cheese sauce.

➤ Serve baked potatoes topped with sour cream, bacon bits, grated cheese, cottage cheese.

➤ Dip fresh vegetables in cottage cheese or sour cream dips.

➤ Stuff celery sticks with cream cheese. Add sliced black olives or grated carrots.

➤ Stuff celery sticks with peanut butter and top them with raisins.

Milk, Cheese, Yogurt

➤ Select whole milk.

➤ Select full-fat cottage cheese, yogurt, cream cheese, and sour cream products.

➤ Make dips by blending cottage cheese or cream cheese with yogurt or sour cream. Season with herbs or seasoning packets.

➤ Make puddings with whole milk. Top with banana slices, chocolate chips, raisins, or whipped cream.

➤ Create sundaes with ice cream or frozen yogurt and various toppings, such as chocolate, caramel, fruit sauce, nuts, coconut, candy-coated chocolates, crushed candy bars, whipped cream, cookie crumbs.

➤ Add powdered milk to shakes and smoothies.

Meat, Poultry, Fish, Eggs, Dry Beans, and Nuts

➤ Select full-fat luncheon meats and hot dogs.

➤ Add cheese to meat sandwiches.

➤ Combine various sausages and crackers.

Appendix A

Nutrient Values of Snack Foods

Bread, Cereal, Rice, and Pasta Group

Food	Serving Size	Calories	Fat (g)	Fiber (g)
Angel food cake	1 slice	75	0.0	0.5
Animal crackers	15 crackers	130	3.0	0.5
Bagel (3 inch)	1 bagel	165	1.5	1.0
Bread, banana	1 slice	165	5.5	0.5
Bread, whole wheat	1 slice	60	1.0	3.0
Bread sticks	1 stick	105	1.0	1.0
Cookies, reduced fat sandwich	2 cookies	140	3.5	1.0
Cookies, regular sandwich	2 cookies	160	8.0	0.5
Cinnamon toast	1 slice	115	5.0	0.5
Corn bread	1 slice	105	3.0	2.0 ·
Croissant	1 croissant	110	6.0	0.5
Danish roll	1 roll	250	13.5	0.5
Dry cereal, unsweetened	1 cup	100	0.5	3.5
English muffin	1 muffin	155	1.5	1.5
Graham crackers	4 halves	140	4.0	1.0
Granola	1/2 cup	250	10.0	2.0
Hot cereal, oatmeal	1 cup	145	2.5	4.5
Muffins, bran, low-fat	1 muffin	160	4.0	10.0
Muffin, bran, homemade	1 muffin	210	9.5	5.0
Pancake, buttermilk (3 inch)	2 pancakes	180	1.0	0.5
Pita pocket	1 whole	75	0.5	0.0
Popcorn, unbuttered	1 cup	40	0.5	1.0

Food	Serving Size	Calories	Fat (g)	Fiber (g)
Popcorn, buttered	1 cup	70	4.5	4.0
Pretzels	1/2 cup	90	1.0	0.5
Raisin toast	1 slice	90	1.0	1.0
Rice cakes	1	35	0.5	0.0
Snack crackers, whole grain, fat-free	13 crackers	90	0.0	4.0
Snack crackers, whole grain, regular	8 crackers	120	4.0	1.5
Sports bar	1 bar	225	2.5	4.0
Submarine bread	1 roll	390	4.0	4.0
Tortilla chips, reduced fat	25 chips	110	1.5	1.5
Tortilla chips, regular	25 chips	140	7.5	2.0
Tortilla, corn (not fried)	1	55	0.5	1.0
Vanilla wafers	7 cookies	130	4.0	0.0
Waffle	1 waffle	105	3.5	1.0

Vegetable Group

Food	Serving Size	Calories	Fat (g)	Fiber (g)
Baked potato with skin	1 whole	220	0.0	5.0
Broccoli, raw	1 cup	25	0.5	3.0
Carrots, raw	1 cup	90	0.5	5.0
Cauliflower, raw	1 cup	25	0.0	2.5
Celery, raw	1 stalk	5	0.0	0.5
Cucumber, raw	1 cup	30	0.5	2.0
Peppers, sweet green,	1 cup	60	0.5	4.0
Potato chips, reduced fat	20 chips	130	6.0	1.0
Potato chips, regular	14 chips	145	10.0	0.5
Zucchini slices	1 cup			

Fruit Group

Food	Serving Size	Calories	Fat (g)	Fiber (g)
Apple, fresh, with skin	1 (2-3/4")	80	0.5	3.0
Applesauce, canned, unsweetened	1 cup	105	0.0	3.5
Banana, raw	1 medium	105	0.5	2.0
Dried apples	1/4 cup	50	0.0	2.0
Dried apricots	1/4 cup	75	0.0	2.5
Dried peaches	1/4 cup	95	0.5	3.5
Dried prunes	1/4 cup	110	0.0	2.5
Fruit leather roll-ups	1 roll	75	0.5	0.5
Grapefruit	1/2			
Grapes, green	1 cup	60	0.5	1.5
Melon, cantaloupe,	1 cup	55	0.5	1.0
Melon, honeydew,	1 cup	60	0.0	1.5
Orange	1 medium	60	0.0	3.0
Peach, fresh, whole	1 medium	35	0.0	1.5
Pear, raw with skin	1 medium	100	0.5	4.5
Pineapple, fresh	1 cup	75	0.5	2.0

Food	Serving Size	Calories	Fat (g)	Fiber (g)
Raisins, seedless	1/4 cup	110	0.0	1.5
Strawberries, raw, whole	1 cup	45	0.5	2.5

Milk, Yogurt, and Cheese Group

Food	Serving Size	Calories	Fat (g)	Fiber (g)
Cheese sticks	1 oz.	110	6.0	0.0
Cheese, cheddar	1 oz.	115	9.5	0.0
Cheese, Monterey Jack	1 oz.	105	8.5	0.0
Cheese, mozzarella	1 oz.	70	4.5	0.0
Cheese, muenster	1 oz.	105	8.5	0.0
Cheese, Swiss	1 oz.	105	8.0	0.0
Cottage cheese, 2%	1 cup	205	4.5	0.0
Cottage cheese, 1%	1 cup	165	2.5	0.0
Cottage cheese, fat-free	1 cup	140	0.0	0.0
Cream cheese, fat-free	2 Tbsp.	25	0.0	0.0
Cream cheese, light	2 Tbsp.	60	5.0	0.0
Frozen yogurt	1 cup	305	10.5	0.0
Frozen yogurt, fat-free	1 cup	220	0.0	0.0
Milk, 1%	1 cup	100	2.5	0.0
Milk, 2%	1 cup	120	4.5	0.0
Milk, nonfat	1 cup	85	0.5	0.0
Milk, whole	1 cup	150	8.0	0.0
Pudding, chocolate, 2% milk	1 cup	300	6.0	0.0
Pudding, vanilla, 2% milk	1 cup	300	5.0	0.5
Pudding, vanilla, fat-free	1 cup	200	0.0	0.0
Sour cream, fat-free	1 Tbsp.	10	0.0	0.0
Sour cream, light	1 Tbsp.	20	1.0	0.0
Yogurt, fruit on bottom	1 cup	350	14.5	0.0
Yogurt, fruit stirred	1 cup	250	4.0	0.0
Yogurt, fruit, fat-free	1 cup	200	0.0	0.0
Yogurt, plain, nonfat	1 cup	120	0.0	0.0

Meat, Poultry, Fish, Eggs, Dry Beans, and Nuts Group

Food	Serving Size	Calories	Fat (g)	Fiber (g)
Burrito, bean/beef	1 burrito	300	7.0	7.0
Ham, deli-sliced, reduced fat	1 slice	30	1.0	0.0
Hot dog, reduced fat	1 hot dog	140	12.0	0.0
Hot dog, regular	1 hot dog	185	16.5	0.0
Luncheon meat, bologna	1 slice	60	5.0	0.0
Luncheon meat, ham (11% fat)	1 slice	50	3.0	0.0
Peanut butter, smooth	1 Tbsp.	95	8.0	1.0
Peanuts, dry roasted	1/4 cup	215	18.0	2.5
Pistachio nuts, dry roasted	1/4 cup	195	17.0	3.5
Refried beans, low-fat	1 cup	270	2.5	11.5
Refried beans, with lard	1 cup	350	11.0	14.0

Food	Serving Size	Calories	Fat (g)	Fiber (g)
Tuna, water-packed, drained	3 oz.	100	0.5	0.0
Tuna, oil-packed, drained	3 oz.	170	7.0	0.0
Turkey breast, deli-sliced, reduced fat	1 slice	10	0.5	0.0
Turkey dog	1 hot dog	100	8.0	0.0

Beverages

Food	Serving Size	Calories	Fat (g)	Fiber (g)
Apple juice	1 cup	120	0.5	0.5
Apple-cherry juice	1 cup	105	0.0	0.5
Apple-raspberry juice	1 cup	120	0.0	0.0
Apricot nectar	1 cup	140	0.0	1.5
Coffee, black	1 cup	5	0.0	0.0
Coffee, decaffeinated	1 cup	5	0.0	0.0
Cranberry juice	1 cup	145	0.5	0.0
Diet soft drink,	12 fl. oz.	0	0.0	0.0
Lemonade	1 cup	105	0.0	0.5
Milkshake, chocolate	1 cup	290	8.5	0.5
Mineral water	1 cup	0	0.0	0.0
Orange juice, canned	1 cup	105	0.5	0.5
Orange juice, fresh	1 cup	110	0.5	2.0
Raspberry nectar	1 cup	120	0.0	0.0
Smoothie, strawberry-banana	1 cup	140	0.5	2.0
Spritzer, lemon-lime	1 cup	115	0.0	0.0
Tea, black	1 cup	0	0.0	0.0
Tea, instant, sweetened	1 cup	90	0.0	0.0
Tea, lemon-flavored, sweetened	1 cup	110	0.0	0.0
Tea, raspberry flavored, sweetened	1 cup	120	0.0	0.0

Appendix B

Guidelines for Selecting Snacks

Tips for Healthy and Convenient Snacking

Grains

➤ Select lower fat grain products more often than higher fat choices.

➤ Choose whole grain products to boost your fiber intake.

➤ Choose enriched or whole grain products for B vitamins and iron.

➤ Pack cereal, crackers and rice cakes in single-serve containers for easy snacking on the run.

Fruits and Vegetables

➤ Most fresh fruits are portable and can be stored at room temperature for short periods of time without spoilage.

➤ Dried fruits are light-weight and resistant to spoilage.

➤ Buy canned fruit in single-serve containers.

➤ Pack fresh cut vegetables in zipper-lock storage bags.

Milk, Yogurt, Cheese

➤ Select lower fat milk products more often than higher fat choices.

➤ Buy single-serve cartons of yogurt, cottage cheese, and pudding.

➤ Look for individually-wrapped cheese sticks and slices.

➤ Milk products require cold storage to prevent spoilage and foodborne illnesses.

Meat, Poultry, Fish, Dry Beans, Eggs, Nuts

➤ Select lower fat meat and poultry products and use higher fat choices more sparingly.

➤ Processed meats (luncheon meats, hotdogs) tend to be high in sodium.

➤ Meat products require cold storage and special handling to prevent spoilage and dangerous foodborne illnesses.

➤ Make trail mix with peanuts, raisins, pretzels, and dry cereal.

Grains	Fruits and Vegetables	Milk, Yogurt, Cheese	Meat, Poultry, Fish, Dry Beans, Eggs, Nuts
Key Nutrients			
Carbohydrates	Carbohydrates	Protein	Protein
Fiber	Fiber	Carbohydrates	Vitamin B^{12}
B-complex vitamins	Vitamin A	Riboflavin	Folic acid
Iron	Vitamin C	Calcium	Iron
	Trace minerals	Phosphorus	Zinc
Lower Fat and/or Lower Calorie Choices			
Bagels		Nonfat or 1%	Fat-free refried
Bread and rolls	Dried, fresh, or	milk	beans
Dry cereal	canned fruit	Fat-free cream	Baked beans
Popcorn, unbuttered	Fresh, frozen, or	cheese*	Reduced fat or lean
Pretzels	canned vegetables	Reduced fat	luncheon meats
Reduced fat or fat-	Fruit juice	cheeses; nonfat	Reduced fat hotdogs
free cookies and		milk cheeses	Turkey breast
crackers		Low-fat or nonfat	Lean roast beef
Rice cakes		cottage cheese,	and ham
		yogurt, frozen	Turkey ham or
		yogurt, and ice	turkey dog
		cream	
		Pudding made	
		from nonfat	
		or 1% milk	
Higher Fat and/or Higher Calorie Choices			
Chips and cheese	Avocados	Cheese	Hot dogs
curls	Creamed	Whole milk	Luncheon meats
Cookies	vegetables	Regular cottage	Nuts
Croissants	Olives	cheese	Peanut butter
Pastries		Regular yogurt	Peanuts
Snack crackers		Ice cream	Pepperoni
			Refried beans
			Sausage

*Regular and reduced-fat cream cheese are in the Fats and Oils Group; however, fat-free cream cheese has a higher protein and calcium content, so it can be classified in the Milk Group.

Appendix C

Satisfying Sensory Cravings:
Lower Fat and Lower Calorie Choices

Chewy
Chewing gum
Dried fruit (raisins, apricots,
   peaches, prunes)
Fig bars

Fruit leather roll-ups
Fruit-flavored chews
Gummy candies
Licorice

Crunchy
Apple
Baked or low-fat snack chips
Bread sticks
Low-fat crackers

Popcorn
Pretzels
Raw vegetables (carrots, celery,
   cauliflower, broccoli)

Sweet
Angel food cake
Animal crackers
Applesauce
Fig bars
Frozen juice bars or popsicles
Frozen yogurt, low-fat
Fruit (fresh, dried, canned)

Graham crackers
Pudding
Sandwich cookies
Sugar-free jam/jelly on toast,
   English muffin, or bagel
Vanilla wafers

Salty
Baked or low-fat chips
Bread sticks
Low-fat crackers

Popcorn
Pretzels
String cheese

Thirst-Quenching

Frozen juice bar or popsicle
Fruit juice spritzers
Mineral Water

Sparkling water
Tap water
Vegetable juice

Cold

Frozen banana
Frozen juice bar or popsicle
Fruit slush
Low-fat frozen yogurt or ice cream

Pudding shake
Smoothie
Sorbet

Hot

Bean burrito (made with fat-free
  refried beans)
Coffee
Herbal tea
Hot cereal
Hot chocolate
Low-fat hot dog

Pancake/waffle
Popcorn
Soft pretzel
Soup
Tea
Toast
Toasted bagel or English muffin

Index

electrolytes, 43
emotions, 2–3
evening snacks, 66–67
exercise (see athletics)

fast food, 74–75
fat intake, children and, 17–18
fat, dietary
  calories and, 11–12
  carbohydrates and, 40
  weight gain and, 79
fat-containing foods, digestion of, 7
fiber-containing foods, digestion of, 7
finger foods, children and, 21–22
fitness (see athletics)
fluids, 34
  air travel and, 75
  athletics and, 41, 43
  weight loss and, 51–52, 54
Food Guide Pyramid, 4–6
food allergy, 22
food groups, serving recommendations, 5
food intolerance, 22
food, effect on heart, x

girls, teenaged, choosing snacks, 32
grazing, definition of, ix

heart disease, 30
heartburn, x
home, snacking at, 65–69
hors d'oeuvres, 68
hunger, 2, 7, 11, 51–52
  athletics and, 42
hyperactivity, sugar and, 12, 14
hypoglycemia, 78–79

infections, 41
intolerance, food, 22
introducing new foods, children and, 22